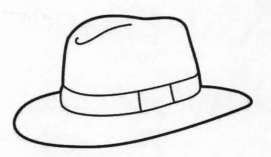

Wear a Hat

The Concussion Recovery Lifestyle

Jonathan B Smith, DC, CSCP

ISBN

Paperback   979-8-9891-4080-0
EPUB   979-8-9891-4081-7
Audiobook   979-8-9891-4082-4

Library of Congress Control Number 2023921745

Published by Jonathan B. Smith, DC
San Rafael, CA

Cover design by Keenan
Editing by Anne Cole Norman

Book Intent and Disclaimer

The content of this book is meant to inform the reader and is not meant to be used as a substitute for professional guidance by an accredited health care practitioner. It is not meant to diagnose, treat, cure or prevent disease. Nor should the information herein be considered the rendering of medical, psychological, legal or spiritual services. Please seek the counsel of those professionals in those areas of service for guidance specific to your individual needs.

While it is the intent of the author and publisher to present the most comprehensive, up to date and scientifically established information available, all information presented is based on the personal and clinical experience and study of the author. As such there is no warranty or representation made as to the completeness or accuracy of the contents. All statements, particularly those regarding nutritional supplements, have not been evaluated by the Food and Drug Administration. Any use of the information presented in this book is at the discretion of the reader and liability for any damage, misuse or loss of said information occurring directly or indirectly, including the failure to seek and take medical advice, is disclaimed by the author and publisher.

Statements regarding supplements have not been evaluated by the Food and Drug Administration. Supplements are not intended to diagnose, treat, cure or prevent disease and should not be used in place of or delay medical treatment.

DEDICATION

I dedicate this book to my wife, Keiko and son Dean who loved me and stood by me even when I did not know my self. Thank you.

Table of Contents

Preface

"The whole point of writing something down is that your voice will then carry for thousands of miles, whereas in direct conversation it fades at a hundred paces."— Matteo Ricci 1606.

This book is written for all head injury sufferers and their supporters. It's the book I wish I had when I was first injured. It's easy to read, it's workable, it's simple. There is some anatomy and physiology, but just enough to help you understand the practical matters.

Everything here is from my experience, books, articles, and seminars, and patients I have treated in my chiropractic, functional medicine practice. I have tried to give credit where credit is due.

If you have a head injury, your experience will be different from others in severity and symptoms but similar in the basics. Not everything in this book will apply to you. There are many books on how to cope with head injury, but few on how to heal. I hope this book can give you some of both.

If you care about or for a head injured person, I hope that in reading this, you may grow in compassion and have more peace. If you are head injured, I hope that this book will give you some of the understanding, hope, and guidance you need to lead a fuller life.

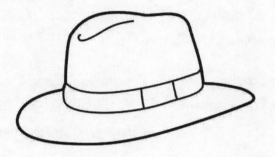

Part 1

Why I wrote this book

There are many degrees of head injury, ranging from a slight bump on the head that makes you dizzy to a potential fatal injury. I had two concussions, the second one before I had recovered from the first. This is called <u>second impact syndrome</u>. Even though both injuries were minor, the second greatly increased my symptoms and made them last.

Since then, I've had two car accidents, been hit by a van as a pedestrian, had two overly forceful neck adjustments from osteopaths and been shaken hard by someone who thought they were expressing love. And then there were all those times I bumped my own head. I now have <u>post-concussion syndrome</u>. You may have that too. The basic definition is concussion symptoms lasting beyond ten days, but we know it means a lot more than that.

My injuries would be considered <u>Mild Traumatic Brain Injury (mTBI)</u>. Even though I know how severe a brain injury can be, I would never have called my own issues mild. When first injured, I did everything I could think of to recover. The problem was, I could not think. I went to many health professionals. I must have gone to the wrong ones. Several told me there was nothing to be done, that the symptoms would resolve on their own over time.

I was told I'd get better in time with no guidance on how to shorten that time. I don't believe that anyone understood my injury. There may have been a neurologist who understood, but she talked fast in terms I did not understand. I just walked out confused.

I remained confused and my symptoms were ongoing, but I didn't give up. I tried to read books, but it was hard to read. Nothing entered my brain. It made me tired and frustrated. The most disappointing part was that I couldn't find any practical advice. There may have been good advice in some of those books, but it was lost in medical language, or fluff. My injured mind could not pull out what to do.

After twelve years of fruitless effort and my multiple re-injuries, I got an email advertising a continuing education seminar entitled Brain Injury and Neurodegeneration. The seminar itself was a presentation of about seventy-five research articles on the topic with very little synthesis of the material into a bigger, actionable picture. It took my concussed brain about two months to create that picture. I took out seven different colored Sharpie markers and a huge piece of drawing paper. I drew lines representing all the inflammatory chemical pathways and noted how different supplements affected them. Then I purchased many, many supplements and took them for at least three months. At that point my head started to clear; I could do more research, and I also sought out more seminars. I still do that.

After 13 years of suffering from post-concussion syndrome and several years of actual healing, I believe it is not just my mission to help other people with post-concussion syndrome, it is my purpose. No one with concussion or post-concussion syndrome should have to wander in confusion as long as I did to find answers. I have shifted my chiropractic practice to a concussion consultancy; the True Brain Concussion Center, (www.yourtruebrain.com). To help you find other practitioners who treat concussion, I started an organization of such people: www.concussionprofessionals.com. Designed to create local groups of practitioners who can work together, the site is divided by specialty, representing all pieces of the concussion treatment puzzle.

In this book, I explain what you need to do to recover from head injury. I cover the most important first steps: mindset, lifestyle, and controlling brain inflammation. There is more that can be done as you progress, but I believe it's best to start with these three.

My advice isn't a substitute for individualized professional guidance; however, I will note that the methods and strategies included here were the only way I was able to heal. The book is intended to be a framework that will enable you to heal, as well. As with all things medical, there is no guarantee.

Hopefully this book will help you understand which pieces you need, though there may be more that are not on the site. If you can't find someone close by, some offer tele-health; you could search by that. If you have a local practitioner you would like to share, please let them know about the group or contact me through the site so others may find them. At this point, the group is just getting started, but I hope for ongoing growth.

Awareness of the seriousness and treatment of concussion and post-concussion syndrome is growing, although I believe there is a long way to go. Many people never seek care or stopped seeking it when given the prescription of rest and time. For some that may be enough, but there is much more that can be done. I hope this book helps you on your road to recovery.

.

Chapter 1

How to Use This Book

This book is meant to be used as a workbook, with short chapters that are accessible to anyone with a mild traumatic brain injury. It's not an instruction manual that must be read in sequence, and it's definitely not a novel, to be read cover to cover. It's more of a reference book that you can dip into as needed, reading the chapters and sections that are most useful to you, and that you can handle, in any given moment.

As your condition changes over time, you can return to the book to re-read it or read it more deeply. As you heal, you may find that some parts of the book have become more relevant to you.

Each chapter is divided into these sections:

- Summary

- What to Do

- Why

- Personal Reflections

- Science and Specifics

Here's an example:

Summary

The summary comes first so the chapter's main concept is immediately clear; you won't need to figure it out as you go along. Once you have the concept, you have a context for the rest of the chapter. Also, if there is a specific symptom or situation the chapter applies to, it will be noted here. If it does not apply to you, **skip the chapter**.

What to Do

These are the action steps.

Read through this part at your own pace; if you don't understand it on first reading, read it again. Highlight what you want to remember or re-read later.

Take notes in the margins on how the material relates to you. Date those notes so that later, after you've taken action, you can look back and see change.

Only read as far as you feel comfortable reading. If you are fatigued after reading the "What to Do" section, put the book down. Do what's most important for you, now.

Why

This is the benefit of the "What to Do" section.

You may find that you do not need this benefit. You may need it, but you need something else first. If so, move on. You can always return to this section later. We can only benefit from what we can understand and use in the moment.

Healing is a process. Your healing process will have similarities to others' processes, but overall, it will be unique to you.

Note that as part of your healing process, your capacity to take in and use information may change. Your endurance for mental activity may become stronger. Your desire to understand may become stronger. This is good progress, although it's important that you don't push yourself too hard.

Personal Reflections

This is the only section that might be entertaining, inspirational, or humorous. There is no guarantee it will be any of those. I used to be a funny guy. I've gotten a little of that back.

Here you will find my commentary on the chapter's topic. I hope that it will add to your understanding of what you need to do to heal, but it will be the least practical part.

If you skip it, you will not hurt my feelings. You may be better off going on to more practical information in other chapters. While I can't promise literary greatness, if your experience of reading or your motivation to heal is enhanced by personal experiences, opinions, inspiration, or humor, look for it here.

Science and Specifics

Here is where you will find more scientific information or details.

If you are a practitioner or, like me, you need to understand something on a deeper level before accepting it, this section is for you. If your brain is fatigued or you have trouble reading, you can safely skip this section.

To make the book more practical and easier to read, technical explanations are as brief and simplified as possible. There may be some technical info in other sections, but most of it will be found in this section.

I repeat important concepts throughout the book. Don't worry that you're missing something if you skip a chapter or a part of a chapter. If you skip part, just make a note in the contents or on that page if you want to go back later.

Chapter 2

A Note on Concussion in General

The distinction between concussion and post-concussion syndrome is one of time. Having symptoms past ten days is considered post-concussion syndrome. Statistics show that 20% - 64% (depending on what you read[1]) of concussion patients become post-concussion syndrome patients. It's very difficult to predict who will be in that group. Both concussion and Post-concussion Syndrome are considered Mild Traumatic Brain Injury (mTBI) in the overall category of head injury.

There are some predisposing factors for ongoing symptoms that are recognized by the medical profession:

11

- Seizure disorders
- Depression
- Anxiety
- Migraine
- ADD or ADHD
- Injuries when the head has been hit more than once
- More than one concussion, especially when the next happens before the previous one has healed. This is called Second Impact Syndrome.

It's my belief that if on some level you had any of the following issues before your injury, your symptoms are worse.

We'll be looking at them more later, but they include:

- Sugar dysregulation
- Thyroid issues
- Adrenal fatigue, severe stress
- Food intolerance, especially to gluten
- Alcohol or drug abuse
- Chemical sensitivities
- Auto-immune issues

- Poor cardiovascular health

Note, concussion can also *create* most of these, except for poor cardiovascular health.

I believe there is a lot of lost opportunity to heal if someone is told to rest and wait it out. The longer symptoms go on, the more complicated the situation can become. If everyone who had a concussion took some of the basic steps in this book, I believe a much smaller percentage of people would get post-concussion syndrome. If you are reading this, you may already have it. Know that you may not have to stay there or at least, it doesn't have to be as bad as it is now. Some of what's written here may be irrelevant to you, but what is relevant may just change your life.

Chapter 3

Why "Wear a Hat"?

Summary

Here I explain why I chose the title, *Wear a Hat*, and why wearing a hat is a good idea if you have post-concussion syndrome. This chapter will be helpful for people who keep bumping their head.

What to Do

Buy a hat. Wear it. I recommend a fedora. You can get away with a fedora inside and out. They look good on men and women. Any hat with a brim that goes all the way around will do.

Why

Three reasons:

1. You will bump your head less, as the brim acts as an antenna. It touches whatever you are about to bump before you bump. You will feel that and reflexively pull back. If you wear your hat enough, it will be like part of your head. You will automatically allow space for the hat when moving.

2. Other people will be less likely to touch your head.

3. If you wear a silly hat, people will smile at you and that feels good.

Why call the book, *Wear a Hat*? Because it's one of multiple simple lifestyle changes that will bring you closer to health.

Personal Reflections

In the weeks following my head injuries and after every exacerbation, I found that I would hit my head on just about any random thing around me. I no longer knew where my head was in space. There was a failure someplace in the apparatus that takes in — and keeps tabs on —one's periphery. Never having been conscious of that ongoing function, it was hard to recognize it was missing. Once I did, it was a revelation to me. I realized I had to expand my awareness of my surroundings and keep that awareness more conscious. I wore a hat.

The idea came to me at a thrift store. After donating some clothes, I was walking around checking out the 8-track tapes and broken toasters when I saw an old felt fedora.

I tried it on. It fit quite nicely. It was soft. I could see the brim in front of me. The crown of the hat and the brim all around felt like radar around my head. This was the best fifty cents I ever spent.

I can't tell you how many times the top or side of that hat hit something before my head did. Just having it on increased my awareness of what was near my head. It saved me countless little jolts to my bruised and tender brain. I wore it inside where all the hazards are and wore it outside mostly so I wouldn't forget to take it with me. It also kept the sun out of my eyes and the rain off my head. In the winter, I wore a fleece pork pie hat. It looked like a short top hat. This had the added benefit of making people smile at me. I highly recommend that you too, wear a hat.

Science and Specifics

If you are brain injured, you may not be perceiving your surroundings or where you are in space well. Your brain constantly processes volumes of information unconsciously. When your brain is hurt, it may not be able to do this well. Part of our unconscious awareness is our sense of our body's position and where we are in space. This is called proprioception and has a lot to do with balance. Our brains also unconsciously process our surroundings. These two work together. Think of stepping over a rock on the sidewalk or ducking under a branch. We do that automatically.

The input for proprioception comes from our eyes, our inner ears, and our weight-bearing joints, muscles, and tendons. Proprioception is organized and interpreted in the cerebellum, right above the brain stem near the base of the skull. Balance and proprioception are closely related. If you are having trouble with balance, you are having trouble with proprioception.

Input regarding our surroundings/environment comes from all of our senses, including proprioception. If you have deficiencies in any of the senses or your brain is just tired and not processing info quickly, you may be prone to bumping into things.

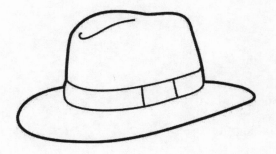

Part 2

The Essentials

Summary

These are your first priorities, the steps you need to slow down, stop nerve damage, and get into the healing frame of mind.

What to Do

- Seek medical attention
- Get support
- Set goals and make plans
- Rest
- Understand your symptoms
- Know your level of inflammation
- Oxygenate your brain

Why

If you've had a concussion, you've experienced an earthquake in your skull. The power grid is crippled. Water and sewer pipes are compromised. Structural damage abounds. There is a raging fire everywhere, creating chaos and preventing clean-up and rebuilding.

In any disaster, there is a triage of priorities. What comes first, what can wait, and what depends on other issues being resolved. A few conditions need to be established as foundational. Consider this section your guide to laying out the basics of your own Emergency Management Plan.

Personal Reflections

My first concussion wasn't bad, but if I'd handled it better, the second might not have been so horrible. The first one happened when I hit heads with another fellow in a martial arts class. I was falling down, he was rolling up. Afterwards, he mentioned that he had a really hard head. I don't know how someone knows that about themself, but he was right. I was startled when it happened, but I felt fine and finished the class. The next day I woke up with a massive headache and ringing in the ears.

The headaches and ringing came intermittently and later on, I noticed I was dizzy from time to time. Certain movements would set it off. I decided I better take a break from getting thrown around on a mat and went to see my chiropractor. At the time, I was seeing a guy who did manual thrust adjustments. I soon realized that this type of twisting and popping of my neck made all my symptoms worse. I didn't understand what was going on so for a while, I did nothing. The symptoms slowly started to go away, but I was still having tinnitus and low-level headaches four months later when I was rear-ended.

At the moment of impact, I was stopped in traffic. There was a split second of black then an awareness that my arms and legs were being thrown up in the air just like those crash test dummy videos. Being in California, I thought there had been an earthquake, but everything else looked normal. I looked in my rearview and a woman in an SUV was waving at me. She said she was playing with her new puppy. I said my neck hurt. She rolled her eyes and called her insurance company.

At that point my symptoms spiraled out of control. Turns out, I had second impact syndrome. Cells in my brain that had been activated by the first concussion reacted more strongly to the second hit. Had I found help and taken the steps needed to heal from my first bump, the next twenty years would have been much better.

The standard of care for a concussion back then — and in many places now — was to just rest. Symptoms would go away in a month, I was told. That may be true for some, but how do you know you will be in that group? Even if you are in that group, wouldn't you rather have your symptoms resolve faster? And what if you, like me, have a second impact during those first months?

We only get one brain, and it doesn't heal the same way as other parts of the body. We need to take any injury seriously and take care of it promptly.

.

Chapter 4

Seek Medical Attention

Summary

The importance of medical attention and what that medical attention should be. This is especially relevant if you were recently injured or re-injured.

What to Do

- Go to the emergency room or your primary care physician
- Get a CT or MRI
- Get follow-up help from a neurologist, neuropsychologist, or concussion specialist.

Why

1. Traumatic brain injury can kill or permanently damage you. It's important to rule out or treat conditions that could do that. Proper management may greatly increase your chances of recovery and shorten the duration or severity of symptoms.

2. Hopefully your imaging will show nothing, but a "normal" CT scan or MRI doesn't mean nothing is wrong; it just means nothing can be seen. If you know something isn't right, you may have to insist on more follow up. Get a referral to a neurologist or a neuropsychologist for evaluation.

3. If a brain injury *is* visible on a scan, it's probably serious. Acting on it, especially in the first forty-eight hours after injury, will dramatically affect your future health.

Personal Reflections

Well you look fine…

One of the greatest dangers of closed head injury versus an open head injury in which your skull is broken, or you are bleeding all over, is that you look fine. You may have been embarrassed when you fell or your carry-on dropped on your head from the overhead compartment. Maybe you were "shaken up" after a car accident, but when the police asked if anyone was hurt, you said no. But you've had a headache ever since, or maybe you're not quite yourself. You're tired all the time or you're overly emotional or confused. But you *look* okay.

If you were bleeding from the head or knocked unconscious, paramedics would have taken you to the hospital. But if you were just confused, or your symptoms got worse later, it's up to you to take action. We don't want to recognize injury. It's scary. Denial may be the most common first response to head injury. Add confusion and poor decision making caused by the injury itself and you may find yourself locked in conflict between sensing that something's not right and assuming "it will go away."

You need to see a doctor! If you were injured recently and didn't go to the emergency room, go now, especially if your symptoms are getting worse. If you're in that situation right at this moment, put down the book and call 911. Or, if you're with someone, turn to that person and say, "Let's go get some pictures of my brain."

Imaging will tell you and your doctor if you had any bleeding or if there's a lot of inflammation compressing your brain. Even if it's been months since your injury, it's good to know. The best news you can get is that they can't see anything.

If nothing is visible on the scan, you can put your mind at ease knowing that the really severe issues have been ruled out. Also, you are now in "the system." You should be referred to a neurologist or neuropsychologist for further evaluation if you haven't been already.

Science and Specifics

The type of scan that's done depends in part on how long it has been since the injury. Within forty-eight hours of injury, the standard scan is CT. CT is faster than MRI and better at picking up fractures and bleeds in the early phase of injury.

After two or three days, the composition of a bleed changes and is more visible on MRI. Nerve damage and brain bruises that come from the slow bleeding of smaller blood vessels are also easier to see on MRI. (Although, note that if you are having a brain bleed, you will know something is very wrong and will be rushed to a hospital, not consulting this book for scan guidance. Doctors will decide what you need.)

Two other types of brain scans are the SPECT and PET. Neither is generally used in emergency situations. They are expensive, not very commonly available, and require an injection of a radioactive tracer to create images.

SPECT and PET show brain activity. Lack of activity in certain areas corresponds to certain symptoms. Like a neuropsychological evaluation, this information can be useful in guiding later rehabilitation.

Chapter 5
Get Support

Summary

Two heads are better than one, especially if one of them is hurt. This chapter is especially for those with executive function (planning, organizing, prioritizing), memory, or brain fog issues. Also very useful for people helping a head-injured friend or loved one.

What to Do

Find one or two reliable people to help you manage your recovery.

Why

Even without a head injury, it can be hard to recognize our own needs and know what to do about them. It's important to seek out someone who can help you with the initial steps of gathering and organizing information. Once you have all the basics laid out—your symptoms, which doctor(s) you should see, etc., your support person can help you make a plan and stick to it.

Personal Reflections

In my own recovery, I failed miserably at getting help, from either a support person or a health practitioner. I didn't know how bad my problems were and I tried to manage my own treatment. I knew I'd hurt my brain, but no one ever said that having a hurt brain makes it difficult to figure out how to heal a hurt brain.

Having a brain injury makes it difficult to organize your care — this is one area where a support person is critical. What is disorganized care? When you're seeing multiple practitioners and no one is steering the ship. Head injury treatment has to be inter-disciplinary; there are different areas of specialty that can affect any one person's recovery. The problem is that each practitioner can be limited to seeing the issue only through the lens of their own specialty. You may view their treatment as the one thing that will heal you, but this is never the case; each treatment is just one piece of your overall recovery. A support person will help you manage your care by keeping the big picture in mind and striking the right balance between treatments.

A balance of care is important, as is choosing the right providers. Unless you or your support person has vast, current concussion education and can quiz your potential practitioner on their own body of knowledge, your decisions are either educated guesses or based on feelings. Who you pick will be the person you trust the most.

But first you and your support person need to ask, why do we trust this person? Is it because they are super nice and compassionate? Is it because they are critical of other therapies so theirs must be the best? Is it because they have an impressive office, fancy machinery, a test that proves you need their therapy? Do they have a lot of followers on social media? Did your lawyer tell you that you had to see them? Are they the first person to offer you hope?

Because your support person is not as emotionally invested and has better brain function, they may be able to help you determine if you're trusting your practitioners for the right reasons. That trust should be based on their level of knowledge and desire to do everything in your best interest, including recommending other people to work with you as needed.

We live in a world that values independence. The message is, the strong are able to take care of themselves. Let me tell you, the truly strong are able to see when they need help and then ask for it. Don't let pride or embarrassment or confusion get in the way. If the first person you ask can't or won't help, ask another. Once it's done and you are getting even just a little help, you will wonder why you didn't ask earlier.

Science and Specifics

For your support person, reach out to someone who cares about you. Spouses, children, and parents may be too emotionally invested to be objective, so choose wisely. A trusted friend, someone who cares about you but could be more objective than a family member — might be a better choice.

Let your potential support person know that you have an injury and need another perspective. Be clear that you don't expect them to solve the problem; rather, you're just looking for someone to listen and help you find direction.

Sit with your support person (SP) and tell your story. Explained what kind of issues you've noticed about yourself. Your SP may have seen changes in you that you haven't noticed. Try to listen without reacting. There is no need to be defensive or ashamed. You are hurt and you need help healing. Both of you can take notes. This alone can be therapeutic.

Have your SP read this book. Make a plan together on how you'll find the help you need. Meet daily or weekly to check in on progress and make changes to your plan. Before an appointment with a doctor/health care practitioner, talk with your SP about what you want to get from the appointment. Make a list of questions. Ask your SP to go with you or record the appointment and have them listen later.

One important distinction: make sure that you both know your SP's role isn't to make medical decisions or steer the ship; rather, it's just to make sure that you stay onboard.

The most important thing your SP can do is listen and understand. Appreciate them.

Your SP is the first mate on the ship of your care, but you still need a captain. The one steering the vessel should be a health care professional, experienced in treating concussion and able to see the big picture. Until that person is found, there is a danger of trying random treatments or therapies that may or may not help you. Resist the temptation to treat yourself. I've seen patients spend a lot of time and money going from one type of therapy to the next without an overall plan.

While searching for your captain, you and your SP need to steer the boat. Unfortunately, this is more like sailing through fog with an extra lookout to avoid icebergs than having a true captain that knows the waters and can manage a crew. You have never treated someone with a concussion. You are not current with the research. Unfortunately, a lot of doctors in this world are also not current with the research on brain trauma.

In your search, you should be asking potential captains, "Who do you get referrals from that specializes in head injury?" That person may be a better captain. Ask how their approach or methods would fit into your overall

recovery. Other questions to ask: *What else can be done?*
Who do you refer to? Their answers will help gauge if they
see the whole picture or are limited to their own specialty.

Once you have your captain, that person is in charge of
plotting the course. You can still use your SP as a sounding board
but he or she will no longer help with *medical* decisions. Check in
with your SP about how you're feeling and for moral support, but
treatments should mainly be discussed with your health
practitioner. If you find yourself reaching out to your SP to make
medical decisions, it may indicate that you do not trust your
captain. You can look at that with your SP and perhaps find a new
captain.

Chapter 6

Setting Goals and Making Plans

Summary

Having goal-oriented plans gives both direction and hope.

What to Do

Put aside time to make short- and long-term goals. These can be how you want to feel and what you want to be able to do. Try to think big picture. Where would you like to be in your recovery and life in a month, year, or five years?

If making plans feels at all overwhelming, reach out to your support person(s) and/or a health care professional that understands the big picture of your current health.

Once you have some goals, break them down into steps and even further into to-do lists. It might take time to figure out reasonable expectations and that's ok — be patient with yourself. Write everything down with target start and finish dates. Put it into a calendar or calendar app. Now you have a plan.

Use your plan as a flexible roadmap as time moves forward. Life rarely goes as planned, but without a plan or destination, it rarely goes anywhere. Always be aware that plans can change. There may be roadblocks. It's also a good idea to have contingencies or at least allow for them. If you don't hit a target, always try to look on the bright side of how close you may've gotten, revise your plan as needed and keep going. Celebrate your accomplishments and forgive any delays.

One of your first goals should be to reduce brain inflammation. Getting closer to this goal will make it much easier to accomplish other goals. About 75% of this book is about understanding and reducing neuroinflammation.

There are many strategies for reducing neuroinflammation; it's a lot to take in. A health professional such as a functional medicine practitioner or a functional neurologist (more on functional medicine in Chapter 32) who is well versed and experienced with concussion can help you with addressing neuroinflammation. Don't hesitate to ask your practitioner questions about it.

Why

When we are not well, it's very easy to go into panic mode. This is both a psychological and physiological response to head injury. In all likelihood, you've never dealt with head injury before. You don't know what to do and it's very easy to become overwhelmed. Stress adds to brain inflammation. Having a plan is really a way to lessen stress. It brings a sense of order to a life experience that feels chaotic. It also brings a sense of hope to a very scary, confusing *now*, creating a path to a healthier, happier *down the road*.

We are programed to forget pain. If we weren't we might never leave the house. We just need a way to tap into that natural programming. Planning and goal setting shifts your focus so that you're not thinking about your pain all the time.

Having a plan also allows you to look back and see how far you've come. That is, you will see the pain you have forgotten. Take satisfaction in that and know that change is possible.

Personal Reflections

Like me, you probably made a quick, immediate plan after your injury. My plan was: go to my doctor, listen to their plan for me, do what they tell me to do. The problem was, they didn't tell me to do anything. They said it would go away. That plan did not work.

I had to make a new plan, so I went to a different type of doctor. In the end I went to many types of doctors and therapists; two neurologists, two acupuncturists, three chiropractors, three massage therapists, a craniosacral therapist, a chi gung healer and a functional dentist. I think that is everyone, though I can't be sure.

Almost everything helped a little, but none of these people I was relying on really knew head injury. None of them could see the big picture and help make a proper plan with me. It wasn't until I took a course on nutrition and head injury that I made my own plan and started making real progress. Taking tons of nutraceuticals wasn't really a plan, though. Like everything else I'd done, it was a desperate attempt to find the one thing that was going to solve all my problems. What it should have been was a critical part of step one in a larger plan. Fortunately, it helped me clear my head a little. I was able to go to more seminars and learn more about the nutrition and lifestyle changes I needed to make to fill out the rest of step one.

I hope this book can give you some insight into the big picture of head injury. It's a much bigger topic than can be handled in one book, but if you understand that inflammation is at the root of many of your issues, you can make a plan. I consider controlling brain inflammation the first step of head injury care and that is what I've focused on in this book.

There are some treatments that help with neuroinflammation; these include neuro-acupuncture and cranial therapies, as found in Cranial Osteopathy, SacroOccipital Chiropractic, and Craniosacral therapy. Approaches that decrease bodily inflammation from injury or immune responses also help reduce brain inflammation. In the end though, lifestyle, including nutrition, is key and that is in your hands.

This book is not meant to be a substitute for guidance from a health care professional. On the contrary, as discussed, it's important to find a practitioner who can help you formulate a plan for your care, and there are many qualified ones out there. A number of them are listed in this resource I created that I hope will help you, www.concussionprofessionals.com.

My mission is to change the concussion paradigm from the rest-and-return strategy to being pro-active about healing. It's my hope that this book and my site will give you access to information and people that will inspire you and help you heal.

After your neuro-inflammation is under control, the next phase of your plan may involve brain rehabilitation. The more severe the injury and the longer brain inflammation persists, the greater the potential damage to the brain and involvement of other body systems. Maybe someday there will be a "Wear a Hat II," but in reality, brain rehabilitation is too individualized to be presented in any sort of guide. If brain rehabilitation is part of your treatment plan, you'll need the help one or more of the following: functional neurologist, neuropsychologist, chiropractic neurologist, neuro-acupuncturist, occupational therapist, vestibular therapist, neuro-optometrist, physical therapist, speech therapist, or psychologist. That may sound overwhelming, but know that help is available. Just make sure you have a plan and that the person helping you make the plan sees the big picture, meaning all of the ways you need help, not just the ones with which they, themselves, can help you.

Science and Specifics

Panic and stress are functions of the Sympathetic nervous system, the fight/flight response. This aspect of the nervous system tends to go into overdrive with head injury. It keeps us in the present, ready to respond to immediate danger. The problem is, there is no quick fix. There are priorities, but there simply isn't an immediate danger that can be changed with an immediate action.

If however, you understand that being in the sympathetic state is in itself a danger, the immediate action you can take is the making of a plan. Once you have done that, you can literally rest, assured that you have done what you need to do in the immediate present and look forward to the paced steps to take in your plan as time progresses.

Unfortunately, planning can be one of the hardest things to do for those with mTBI. It is a part of executive function. This cognitive process is done primarily in the frontal lobe of the brain. If you were in a whiplash injury, your frontal lobe and occipital lobe (in the back of the skull) probably took most of the impact. With generalized brain inflammation, everything is impaired so even getting data to the frontal lobe to be processed into a plan may be too challenging to do alone. Add the sympathetic nervous system, driving you to be shortsighted, and you can appreciate the value of reaching out for help.

.

Chapter 7

Rest

Summary

To recover, both your body and mind need to rest. Rest is especially helpful for those with recent head injuries, flare-ups or brain fatigue.

What to Do

What does it mean to rest the brain?

If you have a cold, you may stay home, read a book, or watch TV. While these things are relaxing, they are not rest for the brain. Reading engages the brain. The way light comes from any screen (TV, computer, phone), stimulates the brain. You may prolong your recovery and feel more brain fatigue doing these things.

Truly resting the brain may be one of the most difficult things to do in our busy, stimulus- based society. The ultimate rest is meditation. In the scientific community, meditation would be classified as Mindfulness-based Stress Reduction (MSBR). Studies have shown that MBSR can improve quality of life for post-concussion syndrome patients and that it increases the grey matter and neuron connectivity in many of the areas of the brain commonly affected by mTBI.[2]

There are many kinds of meditative activities, but they all calm the mind. The simplest form of meditation would be to just sit quietly, allow your eyes to close enough to just let in a little light then breath. As thoughts come up, recognize them and let them go. Correct your posture, focus on your breath or count your breath. This is the way a lot of Buddhist and relaxation or mindfulness meditation is taught. Other forms of meditation are related to different religions. This includes prayer. If you are a religious person and can participate in your religion's form of meditation with a group, that would be ideal. You can have both rest for your mind and quiet social contact.

Meditation takes five minutes or an hour, but what will you do with the rest of your day? I would suggest activities that you find meditative. Maybe you've never had hobbies or pastimes that were meditative. Now is your chance to start!

Here are some suggestions:

Cooking/baking

Cleaning

Organizing stuff

T'ai chi

Yoga

Stretching

Crafts

Fishing

Swimming

Walking

Canoeing/kayaking

Very mellow bike riding

Listening to or playing music

Singing, especially in a choir

Gardening

Avoid anything that's bumpy, requires much thought, or that must be done in a busy atmosphere.

Getting out into nature is very rejuvenating as is being with a pet.

As your brain recovers and your endurance improves, you will need less rest, but you must always be aware of when your brain is getting tired. When it does, take a rest. At this point, your focus needs to be on energy management. Figure out what time of day you're at your best. Plan to do more mentally challenging activities during that time. Learn to recognize when you're running low on mental energy. When you are, take a break or switch to a less demanding activity. Save up tasks like basic cleaning (sweeping, doing dishes, wiping, etc.) or walking the dog for when you are mentally drained.

Why

There is a delicate balance between the benefits of rest and physical and mental activity. Respecting this balance will help nurture you back to health. If you've been recently injured, now is the time to allow yourself to heal. As hard as it may be, you need to put the demands of life aside and know that rest is the best thing for you right now. This is about being kind to yourself.

Personal Reflections

Much of this book is about sharing what I learned from my mistakes. The single largest mistake I made was not resting. The one instruction that's in every protocol for concussion is rest. Sometimes rest is the only recommendation, yet somehow, I missed that.

Before I had my first two concussions, I'd been married just six months and had recently moved my practice into my own space. Everything was going really well. I remember just how happy I was right before I was hit. Once injured, I knew something was wrong, but it was important to me to succeed — that was my priority. I didn't feel I could take time off from my growing practice. I had bills to pay and wanted to be successful for my newly formed family. I kept jarring my body with each chiropractic adjustment I did, napping between patients and spending my money and free time on every type of treatment imaginable. Maybe I would've lost all my patients if I'd taken time off. I'll never know. Maybe it would not have taken fifteen years for me to have some sense of recovery. I'll never know.

Each of us only has one brain. Our success or failure, happiness or emotional collapse, all depend heavily on our brain health. We can always get another job. We can ask our friends and family to understand that we need to take less responsibility for a while. With head injury there's a great sense of loss. If we can't do the things we feel define us, it feels like who we are is slipping away. We fear that if we let parts of ourself slip away, they may be gone for good. It's very hard to understand that if we don't let them slip away for a time, it's more likely that they will be gone permanently. Rest. Heal. Live to be well another day.

Science and Specifics

The brain needs a stable physical and chemical environment to heal and function well. With head injury, both of these are disrupted. Therefore, it's important not to put physical, chemical, or metabolic stress on the brain. Physical stress means anything that will jar or increase the pressure within your head. Chemical stress has a lot to do with inflammation and what you put into your body or what you are exposed to in your environment. Metabolic stress comes from normal activities, such as thinking and processing outside stimuli. To do these things, brain cells need to be healthy and well connected. They need enough resources: glucose or ketones and oxygen. All of these are challenged with brain trauma. It takes time and requires a balance of rest and activity to heal.

When nerve cells fire, they release chemicals to stimulate other connected neurons. After a head injury, the chemical state is one of over-excitation. That means the neurons are easily stimulated. They fire too much and cannot recover properly. They become fatigued. This makes it difficult to think and may give you brain fog. Fatigue with mental activity is called low brain endurance. A good analogy is overworking a strained muscle: if you use it too much while it's healing, it will become even more damaged.

With time and strategies you'll find in this book, your brain's chemical environment will change, neurons will become stronger and form new connections. Physical and mental rest will give your brain a chance to heal. There will be a time to challenge yourself and "rehab" your brain, but not in the days or possibly weeks after impact or if you have low brain endurance.

If you find yourself very tired and easily fatigued mentally, this is your brain talking to you. Listen. If an injured athlete returns to play too soon, they can lose a season. Better to miss a few games. Challenging your brain too soon will make you more fatigued, upset, and maybe even depressed. This slows your recovery. Focus your limited mental energy on healing.

Chapter 8

Understanding Symptoms

Summary

This chapter is for those looking to better understand what's happening in their brain so that they can provide more direction to their healing path. It's also for support people who'd like to see the bigger picture of the recovery landscape.

To comprehend what occurs with your brain in a concussion, it's necessary to examine the injured brain's seven basic problems. They are all related, but you may not necessarily have all of them.

They are:

- Neuroinflammation – when there is irritation and swelling in and around brain cells
- Neuro-excitotoxicity - when neurons fire too easily and get tired
- Nerve damage - when nerves are moved, stretched or broken
- Blood brain barrier weakness - when chemicals that do not belong in the brain's environment enter into it
- Brain autoimmunity - when the immune system attacks the brain
- Decreased oxygen to the brain - when blood flow is limited
- Decreased cerebrospinal fluid flow - when fluid around the brain gets stagnant

What binds these problems all together is neuroinflammation. You will see that brain inflammation is the root of nearly all post-concussion symptoms and that each of the other problems both contributes to and is made worse by neuroinflammation. Fair warning, this gets a bit complicated.

What to Do

Learn the basics of what happens to the brain when injured, how it reacts, and how those reactions create symptoms. Apply this understanding to your own symptoms to help guide your recovery.

Why

The purpose of this chapter is not to have you become your own doctor. However, it should help you choose your doctors. With a very basic understanding of brain trauma and how it leads to symptoms, you and your support person will be able to ask doctors better questions about different recommendations or treatments.

Understanding provides you with context for your different symptoms and therapies, and may also give you a greater sense of control and peace of mind. That alone can reduce confusion, frustration, and stress, which will actually reduce the symptoms you're trying to understand.

Personal Reflections

Being a chiropractor, I knew how biomechanical issues affect nerve conduction, blood flow, CSF flow and even air flow to the lungs before my first concussion. But I didn't know anything about brain inflammation. This is the trouble with being a specialist or seeing a specialist. Sometimes, we only see an issue through the lens of our own specialty and don't see the big picture.

For me that resulted in seeing a variety of chiropractors, osteopaths, and craniosacral therapists. All of those treatments gave me limited, temporary relief, but the underlying neuroinflammation raged on because I wasn't addressing all the factors involved. I didn't realize that neuroinflammation was really the source of many of my brain symptoms. Once I got that, I changed my lifestyle and took supplements to dampen the fire that was smoldering in my brain. That's when the benefits of the chiropractic and cranial work started to last longer.

Each head injury is different, but I do think neuroinflammation is the common thread that links many of our symptoms. I could have named this book Concussion and Neuroinflammation, but who would want to read that, especially with a concussion? There is a lot more to dealing with mTBI than the biochemical, but even if we look at some of the emotional factors, I think you will see how calming the mind or changing how we react has its own chemical expression.

I hope this chapter gives you better perspective on your situation as a whole. Neuroinflammation is a key concept that we'll be coming back to a lot; with so many different possible therapies available, good questions to ask practitioners are, "How does this relate to my neuroinflammation?" If they have a good answer for that, you can then ask them, "What else would you recommend for my neuroinflammation?" If they answer both questions well, you can be confident they see the big picture.

Science and Specifics

Neuroinflammation

Inflammation in the brain and spinal cord is different from inflammation in the rest of your body; it's created by different cell types with different chemical reactions. This being said, brain inflammation can trigger inflammation in the body and vice versa.

Certain symptoms of mTBI relate directly to how badly your brain is inflamed, and that degree of inflammation depends on several factors. The first factor is whether you already had some brain inflammation before being concussed; this, not surprisingly, will make your symptoms worse. How hard you were hit and how long you were unconscious matter. Your general health, diet, and lifestyle also play big parts in how you respond to the initial trauma.

Neuroinflammation impacts our cognitive abilities and emotional state; that's what puts it at the root of the majority of post-concussion syndrome symptoms. The most common effects of brain inflammation are brain fog and unresponsive depression.

The next six problems can both cause brain inflammation and be caused by brain inflammation. Becoming familiar with these conditions can be helpful in understanding how your choices affect your brain health.

Neuro-excitotoxicity

When a nerve fires normally, it starts with a stimulus. A stimulus causes chemicals called neurotransmitters to be released. Neurotransmitters tell nerve cells to let in certain minerals. The minerals have different electrical charges and send a charge down the neuron signaling more neurotransmitter release, which alerts neighboring neurons. After a nerve fires, it pumps out the minerals it let in and is ready to fire again when stimulated.

Part of the inflammatory process involves the release of the neurotransmitters glutamate and aspartate from two types of cells in the brain called astrocytes and microglia. Glutamate and aspartate cause calcium to rush into nerve cells and they fire. Damaged cells have less energy to pump the calcium back out, which makes the nerve cell more sensitive. It takes less stimuli to make the nerve fire, so it fires more easily and often and gets tired. Another way to say this is that the nerve is excited by toxins: neuro-excitotoxicity. Think of excitotoxicity as something going on within the nerve cells.

Symptoms related to neuro-excitotoxicity include:

- mental fatigue
- brain fog
- easy over-stimulation by smell, sound, light, chaotic situations
- irritability
- emotional volatility

Nerve damage

The force of an initial brain injury may have stretched, torn, or broken nerve cells. This will create problems in whatever job those nerves do, including learning, memory, emotional control, balance, movement, sensation, etc.

If damaged nerves die, they spill the fluids that are inside them into the fluid around them, causing inflammation and neuro-excitotoxicity. If the inflammation is ongoing, it can create even more nerve damage.

Nerve damage can be related to symptoms based on the damage's location in the brain. Not all nerve damage is permanent; we can make new nerve connections to regain some function. This is called neuroplasticity and can be achieved through physical and mental brain exercises. Neuroplasticity will be covered more in the next-to-last chapter of this book, "Where to Go from Here."

When rehabilitating the brain to make new connections, it's important to make sure brain inflammation is under control as much as possible. Otherwise, you risk over-working the neurons and causing more inflammation. There is a delicate balance between working the brain to strengthen it and over-working it and causing more damage. Remember, the nerve cells, themselves, have been damaged, and they need time to recover.

Blood-brain barrier weakness

The blood-brain barrier (BBB) is a filter that should only let in what the brain needs. The filter is made by cells called astrocytes and pericytes, which wrap around blood vessels in the brain. Inflammation can weaken the barrier by killing off cells or making the connections between cells leaky. Chronic stress can also weaken the barrier due to high cortisol levels. Alcohol and air pollution harm the barrier as well. A leaky BBB allows chemicals and cells from the blood into the brain that should not be there.

This can create further inflammation and even lead to autoimmunity.

A weakened blood-brain barrier can increase sugar dysregulation and sensitivity to it. It may also cause neurotransmitter problems that relate to emotions. BBB weakness can show up as brain fog or reduced brain function especially after exposure to noxious chemicals or inflammatory foods. [3] Think of blood-brain barrier weakness as something that changes the environment of the brain.

Brain Autoimmunity

Brain autoimmunity is when the immune system attacks the brain. This can happen because parts of the brain have similarities to foreign chemicals the immune system has learned to attack. The chemicals come from certain parts of foods, most commonly gluten from wheat and other food proteins. It's a kind of mistaken identity. If the parts of the immune system that are responsible for attacking the foreign chemicals leak through the BBB, the brain is at risk. The result is destruction of neurons and more inflammation and possible loss of function.

You may have balance or movement issues. You may have areas of weakness or numbness, (though autoimmunity is not the only possible cause). You may get sick a lot or feel a general malaise. You may notice that these symptoms are worse after eating or when you have certain foods.

You can have early brain auto-immunity and no symptoms of it; this is called silent auto-immunity. You have antibodies that cross-over to brain tissue, but there hasn't been enough damage to produce symptoms. It may be a good idea to get tested for the antibodies, especially if you or someone in your family has a history of auto-immune disease. This would include rheumatoid arthritis, multiple sclerosis, Crohn's disease, Hashimoto's thyroiditis, Pernicious anemia, or any food intolerances, especially to gluten. You cannot "un-train" the immune system, but you can strengthen the BBB and change your diet if needed.

Decreased oxygen to the brain

All cells need oxygen to make energy. Oxygen is carried by the blood. Very small blood vessels in the brain can be damaged from trauma, cutting off oxygen from the neurons they serve. If inflammation causes swelling, it can reduce blood flow with the same result. Think of decreased oxygen to the brain as the brain suffocating. It makes every symptom of brain injury worse and can cause further nerve damage from cell death and more inflammation.

With head trauma, the most extreme and dangerous case of decreased oxygen to the brain happens when there is bleeding inside the brain. This is a medical emergency and requires immediate attention.

Decreased Cerebrospinal Fluid flow

There is a tissue called dura that surrounds your brain and spinal cord like a bag. It connects to the inside of your skull and your sacrum at the base of your spine and a few places in between. Inside the bag is Cerebrospinal Fluid, CSF, which is shifted around the brain and spinal column by subtle movements of the cranial bones and sacrum.

The skull is like a 3-D jigsaw puzzle. All the pieces of the puzzle move in relation to each other in sync with the movement of the sacrum. This shifting causes the CSF to move within the dura.

CSF serves many purposes. The simplest is that it provides a cushion between your brain and the bony helmet of your skull. It also serves some of the same purposes as blood. A lot of nutrients the brain needs diffuse into the CSF from blood. Toxins from normal metabolism and inflammation diffuse out. There are also neurotransmitters in the CSF that affect brain activity.

With head trauma, the alignment or movement of the cranial bones and dura may change and affect the movement of the

CSF. Like a stream that has been dammed up and turns into a swamp, the CSF can become stagnant. The nutrients the brain needs do not circulate as well. The toxins that are produced from normal metabolism and inflammation can build up, which creates more inflammation. Think of decreased CSF flow as a slowing in both the supply chain and garbage removal systems of the central nervous system.

Chapter 9

Know your Degree of Brain Inflammation

Summary

There are different degrees of brain inflammation. To understand how to approach your own symptoms, it's important to know where you are on the continuum of inflammation.

What to Do

Get an idea of your general level of brain inflammation based on your symptoms and with the help of your doctor. Below is a quick list of the different levels — for a more detailed explanation, see "Science and Specifics," below. Keep in mind that these levels can overlap. Here they are:

- Acute - the initial period of inflammation. Symptoms may get worse, then begin to taper off within weeks.

- Chronic - when symptoms last and get worse.

- Microglial Priming - characterized by flare-ups and oversensitivity to any kind of brain irritation.

- Blood Brain Barrier permeability - characterized by chemical sensitivity.

- Neurological Autoimmunity - can be hard to detect, may have symptom flare-up when eating certain foods.

- Neuroexcitotoxicity - may be present at any level. Easy over-stimulation by smell, sound, light, chaotic situations.

Why

Once you know the degree of inflammation you have, you can apply the right strategies to lessen it and/or manage it. Sometimes just knowing why something is happening can be comforting. Understanding leads to solutions.

Personal Reflections

There are different statistics regarding concussion and post-concussion syndrome. About 80 - 90% of concussions in young athletes resolve in two weeks.[4] That means they never make it past the acute inflammation stage. You may see many articles that say most resolve by themselves in one to three months. These people have started to develop chronic inflammation and reversed it. A more recent study reports that 54 - 64% of mTBI patients still have symptoms at six to twelve months.[5] That is well established chronic inflammation or worse.

The health care industry has made much progress in concussion management over the last fifteen years. The problem I see is that some concussion protocols don't go beyond strategies for acute inflammation. The primary strategy simply being rest. No matter what level your inflammation, judicious rest will help and should be used. But even if you have just recently been injured, why wait to find out if you'll be in that other 20 - 64% that develop chronic inflammation, microglial priming, or neuro-autoimmunity? I believe that you should be proactive and prevent the next stage of inflammation from occurring, the sooner the better.

Science and Specifics

The brain becomes inflamed or stays inflamed in several ways. While there are many processes and chemical reactions that create inflammation in the brain, (neuroinflammation), there are two types of cells that stand out when looking at what makes one level of inflammation different from another. Those cells are microglia and astrocytes.

When the brain is injured, both microglia and astrocytes release chemicals that cause <u>acute inflammation</u>. The worse the injury, the more chemicals, the more inflammation, the more severe the symptoms. How your brain and body respond to this initial burst of inflammation depends on two things: 1) how well your body functioned before injury, and 2) how much rest, nutritional support, exercise, and protection you give your brain post-injury. Symptoms may include headaches, brain fog, and brain fatigue. You may not be as quick mentally and you will get tired when you are doing something that requires concentration. If all goes well, symptoms peak and then start to fade within a few weeks.

<u>Chronic inflammation</u> happens when acute inflammation sets in motion processes that feed on one another and produce

lasting inflammation. The severity of the reaction may be affected by — or affect — other systems of the body, and can create vicious cycles. Symptoms may plateau, but often snowball.

If you're reading this book, you probably have chronic inflammation or worse, and you're wondering what the heck is going on. Chronic inflammation will bring about the same symptoms as acute inflammation (headaches, brain fog, and brain fatigue), but worse. You may also be sleepy all the time, lose your appetite, or feel depressed. You may find that you "are not yourself." It may be difficult to just think or speak, find words, or make plans. Even going about your daily activities may be mentally exhausting. Your emotions may be out of control. You find yourself confused. You can't tolerate busy situations.

Microglial priming means that microglia cells in your brain have actually changed their shape and function. How scientists describe microglia cells has changed as more has been learned. Now they are shifting toward more specific descriptions of behavior rather than broad classifications. For our purposes, we will use the somewhat outdated but simpler descriptions.

In the absence of trauma, microglia perform many functions. They are very active even though scientists may call them "resting." In acute and chronic inflammation, they would call the microglia cells activated. The more activated they are, the more severe the inflammation.

With severe or multiple injury or other irritation to the brain, the microglia can change their shape and nature. This is called priming. There are two general expressions of primed microglia cells—in other words, they can behave in one of two basic ways. The M1 expression is aggressively inflammatory and reacts strongly to inflammatory triggers. The M2 is anti-inflammatory. Once a microglia cell is primed, it stays primed, however its behavior or "expression" can change between M1 and M2.

With microglial priming, symptoms may become more severe and unpredictable. One mark of priming is that you are vulnerable to flare-ups. You may feel like you're improving, or at least stabilizing, and something happens. It may be a small bump to the head, or you walk by a nail salon and inhale those chemicals and your symptoms spike. You may have good days and bad days and not know why. Something is triggering the M1 microglia or switching M2s to M1s and causing symptoms. This is called sickness behavior.

Astrocyte cells release the same inflammatory chemicals as microglia. Healthy astrocytes protect the brain by tightly wrapping around blood vessels and limiting what's allowed into the brain from the blood. They are a major part of the Blood-brain barrier (BBB).

When the brain is inflamed, astrocytes can be weakened or damaged, creating blood- brain barrier permeability; it leaks. As discussed, this lets in chemicals that shouldn't be in the brain and causes more inflammation. Regular inflammation in the body can also cause the BBB to weaken.[6]

Because the brain barrier and the intestinal barrier are related, damage to either can cause damage to the other. Intestinal barrier permeability is known as leaky gut syndrome. This may result in digestive problems, thyroid problems, and create or contribute to neurological autoimmunity.

The condition neurological autoimmunity, as discussed in Chapter 8, is when the immune system attacks the brain. Antibodies the immune system has created to attack mostly food proteins (that have leaked through the gut barrier) attack parts of the brain that have a similar chemical structure to the food proteins. Once the immune system is programed to make these antibodies, you cannot deprogram it. You can, however, avoid the foods that trigger the program. Because the antibodies must pass through the blood brain barrier to attack the brain, the severity of neurological autoimmunity is directly related to the health of the blood brain barrier.

Neuroexcitotoxicity is when weakened neurons cannot reset well after firing (also discussed in Chapter 8) can go along with any degree of neuroinflammation. Neuroexcitotoxicity keeps brains cells in a constant state of irritability and fatigue.

You may have realized that these "degrees" of inflammation can be progressive. The physiological processes and symptoms can also overlap. This book will present strategies for addressing each level of inflammation, but they overlap, too. It may be wise for you to use strategies that are for the next higher level of inflammation to prevent yourself from going there.

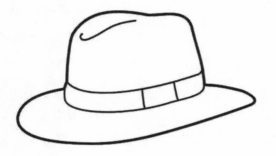

Part 3

Reducing Brain Inflammation: First Steps

Summary

Basic strategies for reducing the cycle of brain inflammation, which is critical to healing.

What to Do

- Take Arnica (homeopathic remedy)
- Apply ice to any part of your body that aches
- Use anti-inflammatory drugs with caution
- Quit
  - Alcohol
  - Caffeine
  - Tobacco
  - Marijuana

Why

Whatever damage was done at the moment of impact to your head is done. So, why are your symptoms getting worse days, weeks, or even months later? Why do you start to feel better, then regress? The answer is inflammation. It's a natural response to injury. No matter how far you've come, controlling inflammation will be critical to your progress.

The next few chapters are meant to guide you through some steps you can take right away to reduce brain inflammation. Note, these are the first steps; there are many other strategies to reduce brain inflammation that we'll look at in Part 6: "What the Brain Needs to Heal."

Personal Reflections

I'm a problem solver. Maybe you are too. For me, to solve a problem, first, I want to understand it. From that understanding comes the solution.

With mTBI, the main problem is neuroinflammation, but there's even a bigger problem: understanding neuroinflammation is a huge challenge, even for people without head injuries. Understanding it on a deeper level and applying that knowledge to your own symptoms is going down a rabbit hole.

I'm laying out these first simple steps so maybe you can clear your head enough to go deeper. Let's agree that in the beginning, it's not so important to understand the problem, so if you'd like, you can skip the Science and Specifics section. Who knows, maybe these few strategies will be all you need to slow the inflammatory cycle. If they do, you can always go back and look more closely at Science and Specifics.

Science and Specifics

As discussed in earlier chapters, the brain has its own special kind of inflammation; it starts with specialized cells called glial cells. One type of glial cells is microglia, which we covered in Chapter 9. Glial cells react to injury by releasing chemicals that cause brain inflammation. Nerve cells become inflamed, overstimulated, and fatigued. This, in turn, can start other chain reactions that create more inflammation, and these chemical reactions feed on each other. They create more and more inflammation and do more and more damage to brain cells. This is why symptoms can continue to worsen long after the original injury. Once the glial cells are activated, it's hard to turn them off and they can become even more sensitive if they go from activated to primed. This is why you may have flare-ups even with slight aggravation of the brain. Controlling inflammation is critical to your recovery.

Chapter 10

Arnica

Summary

If you have a recent concussion, one remedy that's great for inflammation is Arnica, an herbal supplement that comes in different forms. Consult a homeopathic doctor and take the recommended dose of Arnica to help with inflammation. Arnica is best for acute injury, but may still be helpful to take the edge off more chronic inflammation. Have it on hand in case you have a flare-up or re-injury.

Why

Arnica is used for trauma because it reduces bruising and inflammation. A homeopathic doctor may be able to recommend other remedies that are more specific to your individual needs.

Personal Reflections

Although Arnica is usually recommended for acute injury only, I was introduced to it long after my initial concussions and found that taking it for a week made a big difference in my symptoms. It comes in a tiny little bottle that I keep in the basket where I put my keys and wallet every day. I do this to make sure I remember I have it just in case I have a flare-up. It also goes in my "just in case bag" whenever I'm traveling.

Science and Specifics

Homeopathic remedies are based on the principle that less is more and like cures like. That means Homeopaths give you remedies that would cause the symptoms you are having, but in very minute quantities. The upside of this is that if you don't need a specific remedy, it won't hurt you, but if you do it will help you. Classical homeopathy is very individualized so recommendations may be made based on your specific constitution, especially if your symptoms have been going on for some time.

You may have seen this as a cream for bumps and bruises, but it's available in other forms. Diluted tinctures come in liquid form or are absorbed into tiny little pellets. The tincture affects the body systemically rather than a cream, which would be more specific to the area you rub it on.

Arnica comes in different dilutions. The more diluted a remedy is, the more powerful it's supposed to be. For head injury, I've seen 1M or 10M recommended (the M indicates potency), however, these high dilutions are only available through a homeopathic physician. Lower concentrations can be purchased at many health food or vitamin stores. Arnica is good to have around just in case you bump your head again. If you feel you have a negative reaction to Arnica, stop taking it. As always, it's good to talk to specialists about any kind of medications.

Statements regarding supplements have not been evaluated by the Food and Drug Administration. Supplements are not intended to diagnose, treat, cure or prevent disease.

Chapter 11

Ice

Summary

Ice whatever part of your body feels hurt or feels strange.

What to Do

Ice your whole head and neck and anyplace else that you may have been injured. Ice is your friend. If you were injured recently or are having a flare-up, ice aggressively.

For your head, search on the internet for "chemotherapy ice cap" or "migraine relief ice cap." You will find a variety of hats and hoods that can either be put in the freezer to cool or that hold ice packs. I would recommend one that can go in the freezer and is more of a hood so it can wrap around and ice your neck, too. Drape a thin dish cloth over your head and neck, then put your ice hood on for fifteen or twenty minutes of relief. This can be repeated every hour. You may even want to buy two so you always have a cold one available.

If other parts of your body were injured, buy two or three gel packs and have them ready in the freezer at all times. You can buy them in different sizes and shapes depending on your needs. Do not put ice directly against the skin; make sure it's in a covering, and ice the area for fifteen minutes. Let the circulation return to that area for forty-five minutes, then you can come back to it. In the meantime, ice another area for fifteen minutes, if needed.

If you don't like the hood idea, you can go back and forth between the top and back of your head and neck. Most ice packs and the hood tend to warm up after about fifteen minutes, so you don't need to worry about over-icing or setting a timer.

Why

Ice is the least invasive natural anti-inflammatory and pain killer, and it's free!

Personal Reflections

I love my ice hood. Sometimes I wear it even when I'm feeling good; some of the side benefits are that it blocks out a lot of other stimuli. It covers your ears, and it blocks your peripheral vision. This helps your over-excited brain cells to rest a little and may help you focus. Another benefit is that it's like a big "Do not Disturb" sign on your head. It tells your family, "I'm having a hard time right now. I might like your comfort, but let's not have too much chaos."

Science and Specifics

Cooling an injured area does three things. It slows the rate of chemical reactions that produce inflammation. It constricts blood vessels, which can lesson swelling. Finally, it's a natural pain killer, literally numbing the area. Perfect for that pounding headache.

Note that there's a relationship between inflammation in the brain and inflammation in other areas of the body. If other areas of your body were injured when you hurt your brain, it's important to control inflammation in those areas too.

Chapter 12

Anti-inflammatories

Summary

Anti-inflammatory and pain-killing drugs have little benefit for and may even worsen head injury. They may, however, lessen inflammation and ease pain from other injured areas. Since bodily inflammation and neuroinflammation contribute to each other, reducing bodily inflammation may lessen brain inflammation. Always consult a medical professional before using drugs.

What to Do

Be very cautious taking anti-inflammatory or pain killing drugs for your head-injury symptoms. Consult your primary care physician or neurologist on what is appropriate for you.

Why

Studies have shown that over-the-counter and even prescription medications for reducing inflammation and pain are not effective for head injury issues.[7] Frequent use of headache drugs can actually create chronic headaches. [8] This is called medication-overuse headaches.

In a study on rats, use of ibuprofen lowered their cognitive abilities after concussion compared to rats that did not take the drug.[9]

Certain studies show that kids with a concussion who took ibuprofen returned to school or resolved their headaches faster than those who didn't.[10] Based on the fact that the chemical pathways involved in brain inflammation are very different from general inflammation in the body, I am thinking that these kids may have also had other inflamed areas, like the neck, that were giving them headaches.

Personal Reflections

I find a lot of people confuse ibuprofen, (Advil or Motrin) and acetaminophen (Tylenol, also part of Excedrin). Ibuprofen is an anti-inflammatory. Acetaminophen is a pain reliever. Reducing inflammation often reduces pain, but reducing pain does not necessarily reduce inflammation. My personal preference is Advil, and only when ice hasn't worked. In all questions of medication, it's best to consult a medical doctor. There can be serious side effects to even over-the counter drugs, especially when taken often. What is right for one person may not be right for another.

If you are taking either type of drug — ibuprofen or acetaminophen — and getting some benefit, you should know that it's probably addressing other areas of pain and inflammation in your body outside of your brain. It should be a signal to you that those areas need help. You may be able to address those areas without drugs through conservative care such as chiropractic, osteopathy, acupuncture, massage, physical therapy, etc. My personal favorite to reducing local inflammation in the short term is   ice.

Chapter 13

A Note on Self-medicating

One of the hardest aspects of concussion and post-concussion syndrome for me and for others is the loss of control. It feels as if your mind is no longer your own. It also feels like there is nothing you can do. The whole point of this book is to let you know that there is plenty you can do. It takes time and consistency, but you can make major positive changes in your emotional and cognitive wellbeing through lifestyle and diet alone.

In the meantime, that desire to be in control of one's own mental state may drive you to self-medicate. That is, you may want to drink, eat, or smoke something that changes your mental state just to feel in control of it. Of course there are plenty of other reasons one may self-medicate, including escaping from pain or anxiety, relief from depression, social or business patterns, to have a period of euphoria, etc. There is some kind of reward, a temporary benefit.

While self-medicating may be tempting, it's important to avoid putting anything into your body that changes your state of mind. The exceptions may be supplements or medications that influence neurotransmitters or hormone levels, but even these should be used judiciously and under the supervision of a trained professional. And I believe that taking such supplements or drugs should be in the service of restoring the body's own natural balance, and therefore should be taken temporarily, not on an ongoing basis.

When you try to control your state of mind with a foreign substance, it's very easy to get into a too much, too little kind of see-saw dynamic. You never get to "just right." Even if you do, it passes quickly. Tomorrow's "just right" may be more of whatever it was you used, or it may be a different substance to counteract the downside of what you used the previous day. In the end, the substance controls you rather than you controlling your decision of whether or not to ingest the substance, and how much.

Research on the topic of TBI and substance abuse is interesting. Most of it relates to alcohol. What it shows is that a lot of people (59% in one study) who had TBI had alcohol abuse issues before their injury. [11] Intoxication at the time of injury is between 37 and 50%.[12] Many people who have alcohol issues before a TBI reduce consumption for a while afterward, but commonly, they return to their original consumption levels after a time. People who do not have alcohol issues before their injury often develop them at a rate much higher than those in the general population. [13]

One explanation for differences in alcohol use may be actual damage to an area of the brain that has to do with rewards. People who have had TBI prefer small, immediate rewards over larger, delayed rewards. [14] It's possible that those with alcohol issues before injury see drinking as a bigger risk, it caused their injury, versus people who didn't have a problem before who see the short-term reward of getting drunk and don't understand the long-term impact to recovery. Either way, it all shows that people with TBI and mTBI have a bigger likelihood of abusing alcohol.

I would theorize that the same issues with processing reward value apply to other drugs and other lifestyle choices like smoking and sugar consumption. Habits form when there is a trigger that leads to a behavior that in turn has a perceived reward. Even if there are consequences afterward, the reward is enough to get us to repeat the pattern. It's really easy to get into bad habits, especially when the area of your brain that helps evaluate reward is damaged. It's even worse when a bad habit becomes an addiction.

Addiction has both the psychological aspect of reward and a component of physiological compulsion. To be physically addictive, something has to change the way the body reacts to it. Accommodation or tolerance takes place when the body needs more and more of a substance to get a reaction. This happens with cigarettes, caffeine, alcohol, and marijuana, as well as with many illicit and even prescription drugs. Withdrawal happens when you've developed a tolerance and then stop or slow your use, and develop symptoms. Using whatever you are withdrawing from will provide a fix to alleviate the withdrawal symptoms, but it keeps you in the addictive cycle. For most physical addictions, it's best to taper down slowly until you get to a point where you can go cold turkey and quit completely.

The trouble with self-medicating is that you are opening yourself up to psychological and possibly physical addiction. Even something as seemingly harmless as sugar, that provides a temporary boost, can become a habit with negative consequences. The boost is the reward, the lack of energy or crash is the trigger for the next dose.

If you're already in the downward spiral of self-medicating, you need to turn it around. Easier said than done. Start by understanding that whatever reward you are getting is harmful in the long run. There is a greater reward in your future if you refrain. Be mindful of your triggers; they may be very simple, like taking a break from work and having a sweet snack, or more complex, related to deep psychological needs or issues. Recognizing your triggers will help you change. If you find that you cannot change on your own, seek help.

As hard as it may be to resist the urge to "cheat" and self-medicate, we have to realize that the short-term reward is outweighed by the long-term reward, which is letting the body heal. We have a natural ability to heal given the right conditions. With this in mind, I try to put my trust in the body.

The following chapters look at a few of the substances that are commonly used in our society to sharpen or relax the mind. All of these impact neuroinflammation and should be avoided.

Chapter 14

Don't Drink Alcohol

Summary

It sounds simple enough; do not drink alcohol.

What to Do

Again, do not drink alcohol. There are so many reasons this could be a hard thing for you not to do. If that's the case, take a page from Alcoholics Anonymous and go one day at a time. Whenever you have the urge to drink, weigh the consequences versus the rewards. I don't say risks versus rewards here, because we know what will happen and it will not be good.

Do that for a week. Do it again for a month. See what happens. I guarantee you that you will feel better on many levels. Your head will be clearer. You will have more energy. You will be happier. You may feel so good that you think it's okay to drink again. You will be wrong. It's okay to be wrong, that's how we learn. Don't beat yourself up, just start over. If it's really hard for you to stop, get help. Be part of a concussion support group, see a private counselor, or join AA.

Drinking alcohol with a head injury is like trying to put out a fire with gasoline. Your brain is already inflamed and your thoughts scattered. Don't make it worse.

Why

You've had an injury that makes you tired, lowers your threshold for emotional reactions, slows your cognitive abilities, impairs memory, and creates pain in your head. Why would you drink something that does the same thing?

A hangover is inflammation in your brain. That inflammation is caused by the release of chemicals called cytokines. Cytokines also impair the formation of memories. One thing you should know by this point in the book is that inflammation creates more inflammation. You should also know that inflammation is the root cause of many of the symptoms we experience with head injury. So, in short, drinking causes your head injury symptoms to worsen sometimes immediately, sometimes, the next day.

Personal Reflections

Many people, including myself, drink to have a sense of euphoria. We drink to celebrate, and we drink to mourn. There is a very social aspect to drinking and sometimes a business aspect. Alcohol is a great equalizer. You get to forget your problems for a while. Drown your sorrows, as they say.

We do it even though we know it doesn't work. The problems are still there the next day, and we are less able to handle them with our sick stomach and groggy head. It especially doesn't work for problems caused by head injury.

I have to keep reminding myself of this. I get a headache with one sip of wine, or the brain fog and grumpiness of a hangover lasts a week. For weekend drinkers, it's very easy to "cure" that down feeling left over from the last weekend by drinking again. It is a vicious cycle, don't get into it. If you are already in it, get out.

Take a month off from drinking. This may bring you to the point I am at. The point where I acknowledge that drinking has never done me any good and at this point, can only do me harm. The rewards of not drinking are so much greater than the momentary escape. I should never drink again. Neither should you.

Science and Specifics

Alcohol creates more neuroinflammation in several ways:

- Increases oxidative stress
- Increases inflammatory expression of primed glial cells
- Breaks down the Blood Brain Barrier
- Depletes glutathione in mitochondria, causing more damage, less energy production and possible cell death. [15]

Alcohol is so good at creating neuroinflammation that it's used to create inflammation in the brain to test nutraceuticals and drugs that lessen inflammation in the brain.

Chapter 15

Do Not Drink Caffeine

Summary

Eliminate caffeine gradually. This is especially helpful for those with energy, mood, anger, jaw, tinnitus, or balance issues.

What to Do

Slowly reduce your caffeine consumption down to none.

Why

The brain's response to caffeine is complicated. In terms of neuroinflammation, caffeine may help reduce the initial brain inflammation response to your injury or flare-up. However, in more chronic inflammation, it reduces an anti-inflammatory pathway and triggers the release of chemicals that promote inflammation.

Psychologically, caffeine also has a negative impact. It's addictive. It gives you temporary energy, but overall, it makes you more tired. Like any substance we use to control our energy level or mood, it alters our natural regulation. It makes you feel good when you drink it and bad when you don't, and it takes more and more to get the same effect. This creates dependency.

If you drink caffeine regularly and you go without even for a short time, you become tired, and maybe irritable, emotionally down, anxious, and physically tense. Go longer and you may get a crushing headache. It may feel like you drink coffee to perk up or relax, but this is actually withdrawal relief.

The impacts on brain inflammation, alone, are enough reason to go off caffeine. But it also affects hormones, neurotransmitters, and oxygen transport in ways that negatively impact concussion recovery. When you consider that caffeine dependency creates fatigue, and many of the other symptoms of head injury in people who don't even have PCS (post-concussion syndrome), you are much better off without it.

Personal Reflections

My personal journey with caffeine has been an ugly one. In college I was rarely without a bottle of Mountain Dew. This may have been the highest sugar- and caffeine-content drink around at the time. I was pretty wired. I also smoked Marlboro cigarettes, which is a lot of nicotine. Somehow I could get away with this in my late teens.

I went to Japan as an exchange student when I was twenty-four. The Japanese have a custom of offering tea or coffee whenever someone comes to visit. It's rude not to accept. There is also a custom to refill the cup before it's emptied, the original bottomless cup. As an exchange student I was driven around and introduced to a lot of different people on a regular basis. There were days when I had ten cups of tea. This made bathroom breaks very important. It also pretty much turned me off to caffeine for quite a while.

I started drinking coffee again when I was in Chiropractic college. Being basically clean though, just a little coffee would make me very animated; too animated to focus on anything. I realized that I was better off studying regularly and getting a good night's sleep before a test rather than trying to put in extra hours with coffee that last night. When I'd go out for coffee with a friend it would always be decaf.

My trouble with coffee is that it tastes so good. When I came to California and did my Chiropractic internship, I stayed with my brother and sister-in-law. Every morning Debbie would make a pot of really good half-caff coffee. What a pleasant way to start the day. Later when I got my own place, my brother Marc bought me an espresso maker. Best Christmas present ever. What could be better than a shot of espresso and a piece of chocolate? At that point, I was drinking all decaf and never in the morning. I don't think I was dependent on coffee for energy, I just liked it.

One of the reasons coffee is so hard to quit is the ritual around it. Even though scientifically we know it doesn't make you relax, it can seem relaxing and stimulating at the same time. I love the bitterness. What a great combo with something sweet after a big meal. It adds to the joy of sitting down with a friend to talk and can take the chill off a cold rainy day. Yes, I love coffee, but it no longer loves me.

My coffee habit changed a bit after my initial head injuries. I was very mentally and physically fatigued almost all of the time and I didn't have enough sense to just take a month off of work and recover. I kept going by napping between patients and drinking my half-caff or decaf throughout the day to stay conscious. At first, I was so out of it that there was almost no noticeable effect. I was still foggy-headed and going through the motions on autopilot. Once I finally started to recover, the coffee would bring up my energy level a little bit, but it also made me much more irritable, especially towards my wife Keiko, who, thankfully, is still my wife.

It took me a long time to realize what was going on. I blamed all my emotional and energy symptoms on the injury itself. Looking back, I see that using coffee as a stimulant was making matters much worse. I noticed that if I drank coffee after 4 p.m., I was more prone to wake up with a headache. I would clench my teeth more while I slept. Having researched caffeine withdrawal, I now know those headaches were also from the blood flow changes that happen with caffeine. I also realized I had the most energy when I was my busiest because I was too busy to take a break to make or go get coffee.

Now that I am fully enlightened and clean (this is a lie), life is much better. The truth is, I still struggle with it. Like I said, I love coffee. The downside of cutting down on coffee is that it makes you much more sensitive. There's a lot of denial and bargaining around any addiction, so I tend to test my tolerance once in a while. I can handle about a shot of decaf espresso every three months. Any more and I'm just no fun to be around.

Science and Specifics

One way caffeine gives us more energy is by getting in the way of a neurotransmitter, (adenosine) that makes us sleepy. It attaches to receptors for that chemical and blocks it. Your brain doesn't get the signal to rest so you remain alert.

These same receptors can have either an inflammatory or anti-inflammatory effect depending on the level of glutamate in the brain. (As a reminder, glutamate is a neurotransmitter that is released as part of the inflammatory process). When glutamate levels are high, activating the receptors creates more inflammation. When levels are low, activation is anti-inflammatory. Blocking the receptors with caffeine when glutamate is high limits their contribution to brain inflammation. But, when glutamate levels are lower, blocking the receptors limits the receptors anti-inflammatory function. [16]

Studies that show that chronic coffee drinking (more than three cups a day) is neuroprotective before a TBI. It lessens neuroinflammation, nerve death, and blood brain barrier breakdown.[17] That means that if you were a coffee drinker before your injury, it may have lessened the potential damage.

If you are in a more chronic inflammatory state, such as with post-concussion syndrome, caffeine may be limiting one of your brain's natural anti-inflammatory processes. It also increases glutamate production, which can create or increase neuro-excitotoxicity.[18]

Caffeine is addictive because blocking the adenosine receptors causes the body to make more receptors. To get the same effects, you need more caffeine. When you have less caffeine, those unblocked receptors go haywire and you experience withdrawal. The withdrawal symptoms of caffeine can include uneasiness, irritability, dissatisfaction with life, sleepiness, nausea, vomiting, nervousness, anxiety, muscle tension, and muscle pains.

Regular coffee drinkers can get muscle tension and anxiety after just three hours without coffee.[19] During sleep it has been associated with restlessness, teeth clenching and grinding. Jaw issues can contribute to headaches, tinnitus, and balance issues, especially if the bones of your skull are not moving properly, (see Chapter 37: Healing the Musculoskeletal System). Caffeine itself also can create ringing in your ears or dizziness by affecting the inner ear.[20]

Caffeine impacts dopamine receptors and decreases GABA production, two other important neurotransmitters. This increased dopamine-related brain activity is connected to the kind of rage that is sometimes experienced by concussion survivors. Caffeine has also been shown to increase PTSD symptoms in studies done on rats.[21]

Caffeine stimulates the release of a hormone (ACTH) that tells the adrenal gland to produce and release cortisol. Cortisol increases the amount of sugar in the blood. Insulin is then released to get that fuel into our cells to produce a boost of energy. Excess cortisol, sugar, and insulin can all increase neuroinflammation.

This same process happens when we are in danger or stressed. If we were actually reacting to danger and had to fight or run away, that sugar would be used. But if cortisol is releasing sugar due to stress or caffeine, our bodies must deal with too much sugar in the blood. This can mess up the way our bodies react to sugar and have a huge effect on your energy level, among other things. (See Chapter 33: Regulating your Blood Sugar.)

A study showed that people who have 300mg of caffeine (about three cups of coffee a day) have higher cortisol levels after their 1 p.m. cup, but people who drink 600mg don't have this reaction. [22] This may show that we build up a tolerance. That means you need to drink more and more caffeine to get the same response.

Another interpretation would be that the adrenals just aren't able to produce the cortisol in the 600mg/day group. You may have heard the term "adrenal fatigue." The idea is that when someone is under constant stress, the adrenal glands kind of wear out. Caffeine has been theorized to have a similar effect to the point that your overall energy level is reduced. That cup of coffee you used to drink to give you an extra burst of energy now barely gets you up to what was once your normal energy level.

Caffeine affects blood flow. This impacts the amount of oxygen available to your brain for regular functioning and healing. If you drink caffeine regularly, your blood vessels will adapt to some degree, but you are still using an outside substance to regulate a bodily function that should be regulated internally. Stop drinking caffeine suddenly and the blood vessels get confused. This is why people get withdrawal headaches and an important reason why it's important to taper down rather than go cold turkey.

Chapter 16
Don't Smoke

Summary

Smoking is harmful to concussion sufferers in two major ways: the effects of the smoke and the effects of the drug, nicotine. The smoke limits oxygen to the brain. The drug is highly addictive, creating a dependency that can disrupt your emotional state. If you don't smoke - skip this chapter.

What to Do

Use nicotine gum or patches in the short term with a goal of becoming both smoke- and nicotine-free in the long term. If you are an occasional smoker or "social" smoker, stop cold turkey.

Why

Smoking anything affects long-term blood flow to your brain. Even without a head injury, smoking has a negative impact on many brain functions over time.

Nicotine is a stimulant. By some measures, people who smoke do better than non-smokers the first couple months after injury. In the course of about a year, however, the non-smokers catch up in areas they were behind in and have better auditory learning, verbal learning, and memory than the smokers. [23]

Nicotine withdrawal decreases neuroplasticity, your brain cells' ability to make new connections. It returns when you have more nicotine. [24] It also turns you into a bit of a lunatic for about two weeks. If and when and how much neuroplasticity returns once a person has quit nicotine completely was not explored in the study.

Those are the neurological reasons for quitting, what about the psychological and emotional reasons? There is a lot of overlap in head injury symptoms and smoking addiction. We like to think that having a cigarette makes us more relaxed or focused, but the reality is that it only does that because once you're addicted, you become tense and unfocused if you haven't had a cigarette in a while. Again, when you're head-injured and your emotions and thinking are inconsistent or out of control, it's tempting to use something to regulate them, but in the end, that substance ends up regulating us. Taking that substance out of the picture will bring you one step closer to smooth, natural self-regulation.

It may just be too much to try to quit suddenly. Quitting creates a lot of emotional turmoil. If you fail, the emotional and physiologic roller coaster you then hop on may be worse than if you'd never tried. It may not even be ideal for a chronic smoker who has a concussion to quit smoking immediately, anyway. Based on my research, I believe it's best to switch to nicotine gum or patches in the short term with a goal of being both smoke- and nicotine-free in the long term.

Personal Reflections

I smoked for twenty years, from age sixteen to thirty-six. During that time, I really couldn't tell you how many times I quit for a day or a month. I know how hard it is to quit. They used to say that stopping smoking is harder than quitting heroin. I doubt that's true, but I wouldn't be surprised if it was close.

I finally quit after becoming a doctor, three years before my first mTBI. It just felt too hypocritical to be helping people with their health while smelling like an ashtray. Smoking dulls your senses of smell and taste, and when you quit, it returns. What I noticed about quitting was that you always smelled the nastiest scents first; dog doo and dumpsters. If you stick with it, though, not only do you start smelling all the good stuff, your food tastes better, too. I might even go so far as to say that you can taste the air and the simple act of breathing feels good. You have more stamina and your mind becomes clearer. The best thing is that you are free from having to plan your life around the need to light up.

In my pre-injury, non-smoking years, secondhand smoke sometimes would smell great to me, other times awful. That thought of, "Maybe I could have just one" would come back into my head. Did you know that if you can actually taste it, having a cigarette tastes like licking the remains of a campfire?

Now I can smell a cigarette from about a block away. The immediate reaction is repulsion. If I get a big enough whiff, I get tense and easily angered. I'll get a headache and that headache will last. That speaks to the chemical sensitivity I still have from my injuries, but it's different somehow. Cleaning supplies and perfumes bother me, but not nearly as much. More like a slap in the face than my head in a vice. There's something very different about cigarette smoke that really affects me, perhaps the nicotine or the many other ingredients added for "flavor" and to help them burn. Whatever it is, even though I never smoked during my head injury recovery, it makes me believe that those who do have to be just destroying themselves. You may be perpetuating some of the worst symptoms you have because of what you are inhaling.

Science and Specifics

While there is some research on smoking and mTBI, the researchers don't all agree on the effects. This isn't unusual in the world of research, but it does make it difficult to know what the best thing to do is.

If you're a smoker, you should know that the longer you've been smoking and the more you've smoked in that time, the less improvement you may have in symptoms. [25] If you continue to smoke, your impulse control may be less causing more risky behavior. [26] You may also have less ability in the areas of auditory and verbal learning and memory.

It's hard to say whether these differences come from the tar and carbon monoxide from the smoke or from nicotine. We do know that long-term smokers have less blood flow to certain areas of their brain. [27] We also know how important blood flow and oxygenation is to brain function and brain injury recovery. Chronic smoking "appears to be associated with" deficiencies in executive function, cognitive flexibility, general intellectual abilities, learning and/or memory processing speed, working memory, global brain atrophy, and structural and biochemical abnormalities in several areas of the brain. [28]

Chapter 17

Don't Smoke Pot (or Eat It)

Summary

Smoking marijuana lessens brain function and negatively affects your overall mood. It also is thought by many to help with pain, but in fact, it does not. If you do not use marijuana - skip this chapter.

What to Do

Just say no.

Why

Marijuana seems to be appealing to concussion sufferers. In a study of college students, those who had a history of concussion were more likely to use pot—and use it heavily—than those who never had concussion. Comparing students with concussion histories, those who smoked pot were more likely to have post-concussion symptoms including headaches and memory issues. [29]

Here's why they had worse symptoms: In the short term, THC (delta 9 tetrahydrocannabinol, the part of marijuana that makes you high) lessens brain function in some of the same areas that concussion does. Some of these effects can last as long as twenty-four hours. THC gets stored in fat tissues and then is released over time. That means if you use often, the short-term effect just keeps going.

Here are the short- and long-term effects of THC. The short-term effects occur while you're high or up to twenty-four hours later. The long-term effects occur after twenty-four hours. Many are reported in studies where people had not smoked in three months to years.

Short-term effects of THC:

- Decreased attention
- Poor executive function[30]
- Anxiety
- Emotional lability (quickly changing mood)

- Drowsiness
- Incoordination, poor reaction time
- Poor short-term memory
- Confusion
- Difficulty doing complex tasks

Long-term effects of THC:

- Short- and long-term memory deficits
- Decreased attention
- Hand-eye coordination issues[31]

It used to be thought that low motivation was a long-term effect of chronic pot smoking, (three or more times a week). Now it's thought that low motivation is the result of the THC just staying in the system. Most people who smoke pot do it for the relaxation and euphoria it provides. Keep it up and this looks a lot like lack of motivation, something that many concussed people struggle with already.

Smoking anything affects your lungs and the blood's ability to carry oxygen. Due to the amount of tar and other chemicals in marijuana, smoking three joints is considered to have the same impact on the lungs as smoking a pack of cigarettes. People who smoke pot regularly are more likely than cigarette smokers to get bronchitis and have lung damage. [32] The brain needs lots of oxygen to function, but it needs even more to recover from injury. Filling your lungs with soot lessens oxygen intake.

Many people use marijuana for chronic pain and may even have a prescription for it. A review of twenty scientific studies showed that marijuana was no better than a placebo in relieving pain. [33]

Personal Reflections

I feel like I've lost a couple people to chronic pot smoking. One was the brother of a good friend in high school. He was in a terrible car accident and went into a coma for about a month. He'd been a pretty heavy pot smoker before, so while he was in the hospital, his friends brought him some food and some pot.

Here was a guy who already had serious brain deficits and his friends helped make them worse. At this point I can never tell if he is stoned or if his slow cognition and tendency to find humor in the commonplace are a result of his head injury. My suspicion is that he is stoned most of the time and when he isn't, the residuals of THC and his injuries make him seem that way. He doesn't work, but fortunately, he has a resourceful family, so he has support and comfort.

I've seen others who were not concussed or head-injured fade away from themselves and their connection to the world from frequent pot use. When I'm with these people, it feels like they're in a different room. It truly makes me sad and kind of angry. Here I am, post-concussion, trying so hard to think clearly and be present, and their choices have made them emotionally absent.

It used to be thought that pot wasn't physically addictive, but the body does accommodate to it. That means it takes more and more to get high. Pot smokers also experience a withdrawal from the drug. Most commonly they become anxious, depressed, irritable or angry. The withdrawal only takes about forty-eight hours, but it's uncomfortable, so it can perpetuate the habit. Moreover, I believe the psychological addiction is stronger and more dangerous — specifically, dangerous to a person's quality of life. After a while, from what I've observed, people who smoke pot heavily tend to stop participating as much in life; they may only socialize with high people and aren't able to appreciate the world as much.

Science and Specifics

THC is a neurotransmitter that affects the receptor called CB1. When you have a head injury and all that calcium rushes into your neurons, your body produces its own cannabinoids that attach to the CB1 and other receptors to slow down the process, thereby protecting the brain. THC also does that. So, there is some benefit to THC.

But here's the catch, it's effective in ultra-low doses, much less than what would make you even a little giddy. That and it's helpful if given forty-eight hours before or in the first week after injury. [34] So, if you happen to walk by someone who is smoking pot and get a whiff two days before or a week after your injury, you can thank them. But that's all you get.

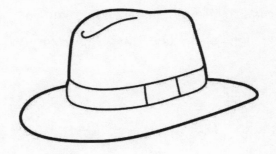

Part 4

Rediscover Your Self

Summary

Brain injury can affect us on a deeply psychological and spiritual level. It can disrupt our perception of ourselves and the world to the point that we feel lost to ourselves. To do the work of healing, you need the strongest emotional foundation you can have. This part will help you reconnect with yourself, interact with the world, hold on to hope, and move forward with a healing mindset.

What to Do

Understand that there is who you were before, who you are now, and who you will be. Know that if you can see that, you have some power in determining the who you will be.

Know that the things you used to do but cannot do now are not truly who you are or were. Know that you have not gone crazy. You have not become stupid. Your neurology has been altered. The way you are thinking or behaving now is not your fault. The brain can heal and find new pathways. Know that you can play an active role in that healing.

Why

Who you are — your identity — is the sum of your private thoughts, your temperament, how you interact with others, and what you do. That identity is the product of time; one experience after another building up to the present.

The brain is the great organizer of all experience. It takes everything you sense and makes sense out of it. It puts it into the context of all your past experience. That past experience contains all your memories, conscious and unconscious. This is the basis for understanding the world and yourself.

Concussion disrupts that connection to past context and how you process new information. It creates such sudden, drastic changes that nothing fits. The continuum is broken to the point that you may not recognize who you are. Loss of identity is very disorienting, confusing, and frightening. Often it leads to a sense of helplessness and depression. Despair can push us to seek relief through substance abuse or even suicide. The real answer can be found in hope and the knowledge that healing is possible.

Personal Reflections

Before my head injuries, I saw myself as a smart, easygoing, moderately athletic, happy person. After my injury, I was stupid, short-tempered, disabled, and tired. This was extremely confusing and upsetting to me. I would see myself struggling to figure something out or suddenly becoming angry or sad and not recognize myself. I had a great sense of loss and a feeling of desperation. I also experienced a sense of shame and embarrassment. I liked who I was before and didn't want people to know I was different. I felt panicked to get myself back, to find the person I had lost.

What I know now is that person—who I thought I'd lost— was still there. When you're head-injured, it's like there's a consciousness of yourself from before the injury watching an extreme version of a tired baby. This poor baby just doesn't know how to process all the stimulus it's receiving. It can't connect with a historical context and it can't filter out what isn't important. It's also just not as smart as an adult. But, as long as we can recognize what this poor child is going through and have compassion, we can help it.

You may miss your old self, or perhaps you don't want to be exactly like you were before. Chances are, you won't be. You are building on new experiences. I may have been too patient, a bit of a pushover before my injuries. During my darkest days, I had no tolerance for even minor things that bothered me, and I would let people know. Sometimes I would observe myself doing this and feel the frustration and rage behind it. It would be like watching a movie and I would think, why is this bothering me and why am I shouting about it? The upside is that I realized people would listen to me and I didn't have to be so accommodating. That part felt good, but the lack of self-control was frightening.

Now, I am more tolerant, but I do let people know when something is bothering me. I'm just more diplomatic and emotionally controlled. My point is that I am not the same person I was before, but that is not all bad. You don't have to return to the exact person you were. It's not really possible, and trying to do so will just be a source of constant frustration. You can, however, have a new self. You may end up being very much like you were before, but you will be changed in some ways and that might be okay.

Science and Specifics

When an injury limits our ability to do something, it changes our perception of ourselves. If a baseball player can no longer play baseball because of a bad shoulder, are they still a baseball player? They may consider themself an injured player. If their injuries cannot heal, they would have to say the words, "I was a baseball player." They have lost something. They're the same person, of course, but they have to define themself differently. In this way, what we do defines us even though we may know it's not who we truly are. We are attached to that as part of our identity. To lose the ability to do something important to us can create a loss of identity.

Brain injury goes much deeper than physical limitations. Your thoughts and feelings may be affected. When the brain is injured, the context in which you interpret what you perceive is disrupted. It doesn't work as well or as fast and it isn't sure what is meaningful and what is not. Even simple everyday tasks may be difficult because the well-established nerve pathway for that routine is disrupted. Some brain cells fire too easily and get fatigued. Other brain cells are damaged or dead. Pathways that dampen emotional reactions may be damaged. The results are many possible different "symptoms" related to how you think or feel. It's confusing and disorienting.

The good news is, the brain has been described as plastic, which means it can adapt. It can make new connections where old connections were broken. This is a healing process and takes time. Most everything we do to heal from a head injury is to support this process. Know that it's possible. Do not despair.

Consider everything in this book as a first step. If an earthquake or tornado demolished your home and the remains were on fire, you would need to do two things before rebuilding: put out the fire and regain hope.

Controlling neuroinflammation is putting out the fire. Knowing that recovery is possible is to regain hope. In the weeks, months, or years to come, you may face many challenges. I challenge you to look back from time to time and see how much you have improved. It may not completely erase whatever despair you are feeling, but it should give you hope that tomorrow can be better.

Chapter 18

Do Something Well

Summary

If you have a brain injury and are having trouble doing things you used to, it's nice to enjoy a sense of mastery and accomplishment by doing something simple.

What to Do

Choose something you were really good at before your injury or something completely new. It should be a simple task, maybe even menial or repetitive. Knitting, doing the dishes, washing the car, making an omelet. Something you have done a thousand times or something you've never done that comes with very simple instructions. It should require very little thought and take about fifteen to thirty minutes or have fifteen- to thirty-minute steps. If you need to, use directions or write out the steps beforehand. Set aside time and put all your focus on doing that one thing. Nail it. Just do it perfectly. Do it again tomorrow and the next day.

Why

This is all about competence. When it's difficult and frustrating to do what was once easy, it feels good to do something well. You will have accomplished something. You will have done it from beginning to end flawlessly. If you haven't, try again tomorrow and enjoy how much easier it is. Let that taste of mastery, even over a trivial task, be a beacon of things to come.

Personal Reflections

When I was growing up, my dad would often make pancakes for Sunday breakfast. It was kind of a big deal. Everyone was happy to have a nice big plate of warm pancakes, some breakfast sausage, and orange juice. My dad was also always happy to make it. Since I've been on my own, I too have been making a nice breakfast on the weekends, first for myself and now for my wife and child. Most of the time, it's pancakes. Before I was injured, I didn't need to look at a recipe to whip up a batch, but then afterward, I did.

Even when I had to read the recipe, the pancakes were just as good and making them and serving them to my family felt just as good. As I learned more about concussion, I shifted to gluten-free pancakes and then again to ketogenic pancakes. I never memorized those recipes, but they became very familiar to the point that I could look at the menu and think, "Oh yeah, that's right," and move on from there.

My sister-in-law loves to bead. So much so she's used her graphic arts skills to create very clear beading patterns. Take a look at https://www.aroundthebeadingtable.com. Not long ago she told me she has had several emails from women who've had head injuries or strokes and she forwarded one to me. Here's an excerpt: "One summer day, I went into the bead shop and told her that I had memory issues and couldn't follow directions unless written so I could track it, and that I had dexterity issues and wasn't sure if I could even feel the needle and thread. She pulled out your Skinny Bracelet pattern. Seeing your printed instructions with the color-coded illustrations was miraculous. It was as if the clouds in my brain had parted and there was some light again. Miss Deborah... to have the opportunity to DO something... and to DO it well after losing so much... to have a function and purpose again... to have a gift to give others... it is YOU I have to thank!!!"

This woman had never beaded before her injuries, but I think you can feel her joy and gratitude at being able to really do something well. Another benefit of detailed-oriented crafts is that they exercise both the frontal lobe and the cerebellum. The frontal lobe controls movement and the cerebellum, fine motor skills. By exercising and improving one function of a brain area, you improve its other functions. In the case of the frontal lobe and cerebellum, she improved not only movement and fine motor skills but also, executive function and balance.

Science and Specifics

The frontal lobe of the brain is the area used for executive function. This is planning, organizing, time management, working memory, (short-term), self-monitoring, and control and sequencing (breaking a task into steps). It's a common area of damage or decreased function in concussion.

When we do something for the first time, executive function helps us break it into steps and put them into sequence. Those steps go into our working memory and keep us on track. With repetition, the steps become connected and remembered more permanently as one task; we don't need to think about each step anymore. This can be disrupted with brain injury — it may be hard to remember how to do simple things. We have to think about each step.

Doing something really easy is kind of throwing your frontal lobe a softball. You are exercising that part of the brain without straining it. You are also creating a reward for yourself. The joy of completing something releases dopamine. Even anticipating doing something that gave you pleasure before will release dopamine. Dopamine makes you happy.

When it feels like so much is just wrong, it's nice to have a little something that feels right.

Chapter 19

Forgive Yourself and Others

Summary

If you've been harmed or feel you have done harm to others, you likely feel negative emotions in connection with that harm. But these emotions will only make life harder for you. Letting them go is liberating and healing.

What to Do

Make a conscious effort to think of the people who have harmed you. This list may include those involved in your actual injury as well as people who simply have not understood what you're going through since your injury occurred. Start with the person about whom you have the strongest emotional charge.

Now is the hard part. You have to find a way to forgive this person in your heart. You don't have to tell them that you forgive them; that puts most people on the defensive, and it could harm what may already be a difficult relationship. They might not think or be willing to admit they did or said anything harmful.

The "in your heart" part is the most important aspect of forgiving the person about whom feel you feel so strongly. If you have emotion to release before you're able to forgive, there are a few things you can do: have an imaginary conversation with the person; write a letter, but don't send it; pray about it, meditate, or talk with a therapist or other uninvolved person. You could even throw darts at a dart board with their picture on it. Whatever it takes to let it go, do it. And then forgive. Once you've cleared your psyche of your feelings about this person, the one with whom you were the most angry or upset, the rest will be a little easier.

Two types of therapy may be particularly helpful for moving toward forgiveness: EMDR (Eye movement desensitization and reprocessing) and CBT (Cognitive Behavioral Therapy). Both therapies are often used for people suffering from PTSD (Post Traumatic Stress Disorder). You may actually have PTSD, but even if you don't, there is a lot of overlap neurologically between PTSD and mTBI.

EMDR uses cues and eye movement to move memories of trauma from a perpetual sense of being in the present to the past. CBT guides you to look at and think through your emotion. You may be asked to consider the intentions of the person you need to forgive, feel empathy toward them, and make judgements about how forgivable the offenses are. You can apply this to your own self-forgiveness as well.

Forgiving yourself may be more difficult. Maybe your injury was your fault. Once you were injured, maybe you didn't take good care of yourself, or you couldn't do your job well, or you lashed out at other people. Look at what you did, said or felt. Understand that you can't change what happened. Apologizing to others for any wrongs done to them and asking for forgiveness and understanding may help rebuild damaged relationships and move you closer to self-forgiveness, but again, the most important part is forgiving yourself "in your heart." You need to let things go.

Forgiving yourself isn't a one-time event, and it's a good practice for anyone to have. As a person healing from a head injury, you may have many opportunities. You are human and you are injured, and you are worthy of forgiveness.

Why

Head trauma can happen by accident, or someone may have intentionally harmed you. Either way, there was an event. You, someone else, or chance was responsible. No matter what, something happened that should not have. That leaves an emotional wound that can only be healed through forgiveness.

Concussion can scramble your emotions. Extreme or inappropriate reactions can lead to feeling that you've lost your sense of self. You may be aware in the moment that your emotions and how you're expressing them is outside of your or anyone else's normal. Even so, you may not be able to control yourself. Repetitive thoughts and feelings of anger, hostility towards others, or shame and confusion toward yourself can take on a life of their own and create a perfect environment for inappropriate reactions in the moment.

The loss of control you feel as a result of head injury may lead to feelings of helplessness and progress to despair, depression, or even self-harm. These are all emotions of fight or flight and keep your nervous system in a constant state of alert. It's exhausting. To forgive is to release yourself from a prison of your own making. You cannot undo the events of the past and the feelings attached to them, but you can leave them behind.

Personal Reflections

Forgiveness sounds easy on paper. The reality is that it's not. Neurology backs up the fact that the more harmful someone's actions are, the more difficult it is to forgive them. The intent is another factor, accidents being much easier to forgive than attacks. Personally, I think there's another factor; the "they should have known better" factor. This one applies most strongly to the people closest to us and the people we seek help from, often one and the same. A health care practitioner implying or outright saying that you are faking or crazy or a family member putting you in a situation they know will be hard for you to handle may be more difficult to forgive than whatever caused your initial injury. Once we are injured, it seems there are so many *more* ways we can be hurt, both physically and emotionally.

I had an interesting experience related to the first person who rear-ended me. This was just a few months after my first concussion. The injury I got from that accident amplified the symptoms I was having and added many more. I was stopped in three lanes of traffic when she ran into me at full speed in a heavy SUV. When we pulled over, she told me that she'd been playing with her new puppy in the front seat and didn't see me. I told her that my neck hurt and I was getting a headache. She rolled her eyes and proceeded to call her insurance company to tell them that she barely hit me and that I was faking an injury. It was quite the opposite; after that accident, I got my first real taste of what concussion was all about. Brain fog, ongoing headaches, difficulty speaking and reading, sound sensitivity, and constant fatigue were all my new friends. The fact that she was so flippant about having crashed into me, and that she gave false information to the insurance company, filled me with rage. Those moments stayed present in my mind for a very long time.

Years later, I was at a body shop. I had been rear-ended again. I happened to look down at some paperwork on the owner's desk and saw the name of the woman who'd run into me years before. The owner was a friend, so I asked her about it. Apparently, this person had bought a new smaller car and boxed in a UPS truck, parking so close that the UPS driver didn't see her car and backed into it multiple times, causing extensive damage. She wasn't in the car, so she wasn't hurt, but her car was disabled for several weeks as they were still waiting for parts.

I had never wished her harm, so I was glad she wasn't hurt, but nonetheless, I felt a deep understanding of karma. Since the accident, I'd felt anger at knowing someone could do so much damage and get off scot-free. But here, I could see what goes around comes around. As a result, I was able to let go of some really negative feelings and forgive her. This insight into karma also helped me forgive others who have hurt me. I don't have to hold a grudge or do anything about it; everything evens out over time.

Science and Specifics

Coming to terms and letting go of negative feelings will literally alter your mind. It will help you shift from being in that sympathetic, fight-flight mode to being in a parasympathetic rest, digest, and heal mode. Forgiveness changes the neurotransmitters that are released in your brain and activity in different areas of the brain. Dwelling on past harm activates pain receptors and releases stress hormones. In contrast, when you forgive, you activate pleasure centers of your brain and strengthen those pathways.

Chapter 20

Know your Now

Summary

To move forward, we need to know where we're starting. That means knowing our state of being in the present moment, including our symptoms and our strengths and weaknesses. We all have unique abilities and personalities both before and after head injury. How each of us heals is different. Use this method to help figure out your own healing path.

What to Do

Start by writing down the symptoms you are experiencing. Then write down your strengths. Write down whatever support you have, everything from your dog to your god. Type everything into a document on your computer, or hand write it, and date it. In a month or three months, check the document, change the date, and update as needed. Do a "save as" so the previous document is preserved. If it's handwritten, jot down a new list. Repeat this process again in 3 months.

Keep a daily journal of challenges and victories. Challenges are times you were triggered or noticed something that was difficult or just not quite right for you. Victories would be those times you took positive steps to prevent or deal with those situations.

Go to a neuropsychologist and get tested. You can find a neuropsychologist through your general practitioner or through a neurologist. You may also find neuropsychologists on www.concussionprofessionals.com, an organization I created in late 2023 for the purpose of connecting concussion patients to local groups of concussion specialists.

Why

Self-awareness is very difficult when head injured. It's hard not to become impatient with your progress, and you may not recognize the progress you've made. Taking time every day to write in a journal about how you're doing, and updating your symptoms, strengths, and support monthly or every three months, keeps you in the present while allowing you to be mindful of progress. This can provide a sense of control and continuity to what otherwise feels like chaos.

Neuropsychological exams can provide an even more objective, quantified read on how you're progressing and provide treatment direction.

Personal Reflections

I started part of this practice by accident. I was going to see a new doctor and knew I wouldn't be able to remember all the symptoms I was having. I created a file called "the condition of my condition." The next time I went to a new doctor, I figured I'd save myself time and just reprint it. What I discovered is that my symptoms had changed! I didn't even remember having some of them. If I hadn't made that file, I wouldn't have seen how far I'd come. I wouldn't have been able to celebrate the victory or gain more hope.

Over time, I'd check the condition of my condition. Sometimes I would have to add something new to the list, but most of the time I would take more off. Looking back, I could see the progress I'd made and that helped me continue moving forward.

Science and Specifics

Some symptoms are easy to understand and explain: You may notice that it's harder to read when you are tired, or perhaps you get confused when you're in a group and several people are talking at the same time. Certain types of pain and challenges coincide with certain activities. Other issues may be harder to understand. You may suddenly get angry or sad for no apparent reason. Perhaps you have trouble expressing yourself on certain types of topics. Symptoms may get better or worse randomly.

Whether or not you understand the symptoms and challenges you're having, it's good to get them down on paper. It makes them somehow more concrete and manageable. It's also very handy for when you go to see a health care practitioner. You can just hand them a piece of paper rather than trying to remember everything.

Acknowledging your own strengths and support may be even more important. You need to give yourself credit, celebrate your victories and be thankful. Sometimes it feels like nothing is changing, but if you write these things down, you may see that they are.

Neuropsychological testing will determine what areas or functions of your brain have been affected by your injury. Great insight can be gained by this kind of testing. A neuropsychologist can also provide suggestions on how to train the specific areas of the brain that may be affected.

Both your own documentation and neuropsychological testing are useful in terms of establishing a baseline or starting point. They can also be instrumental in the creation and modification of your treatment plan. As time goes by, you can refer back to these and see how you have improved.

Chapter 21

A Note on Change

In many chapters of this book, you will be asked to consider a change. These changes might be welcome or they might not; with head injury, it can feel like multiple changes are being forced upon us. We resist and resent them. Thoughts run through our minds: *Why can't we do what we've always done? Isn't the object of healing to be able to go back to the way we were?* Sadly, while we may want to return to how we were, it may not be possible.

But here's the thing: change can be an exercise in letting go. Quitting eating, drinking, smoking, or doing something we enjoy may feel like a loss. However, it's important to understand the benefit we'll reap from making the change. For the head injured, that benefit may be a clearer head, more stable moods, more energy, improved balance, and better memory. A small reduction in any of our symptoms can have a huge impact on the quality of our lives.

Even so, we resist. Not only do we resist psychologically, sometimes our bodies even resist. Emotionally, we long for the time when we could enjoy *xyz*, whether that's an after-dinner drink or a ride on a roller coaster. The feeling attached to what we need to let go of is happiness or escape. We can get to a point in our recovery where we're feeling a little better and think, "Maybe I can try that again." We want that feeling we had in the past. So, we eat, drink, or do again and we pay the consequences. How many times do we have to do something that used to bring us joy, but now brings us pain, before we're truly able to learn and let go?

We can also get pushback on a physical level. Chemically, our bodies get used to our habits, even if they are bad for us. We may be addicted to certain foods, drugs, or behaviors. To change any of these could create a period of dis-ease or withdrawal. It might be necessary to taper down or ease into giving up an old—or adding a new—habit. At some point, though, we need to go all in. Otherwise, we just rock back and forth between the old and new, perpetuating that difficult period of change.

This is not to say that you'll never be able to return to doing things that are actually good for you. Reading may cause mental fatigue now, but once you can ease back into it, you'll find that it's enriching, with the added bonus of building new connections in the brain. Likewise, certain exercises may have too much impact or be too disorienting for you now, but if you can work your way back into them over time, the movement and exertion will benefit you on many levels.

Sadly, we may be best without things we consider indulgences; that daily sweet treat you love, the special wine, an after-meal smoke, maybe even a simple piece of toast. But we have to ask ourselves, is the momentary pleasure worth the setback? Sometimes you're going to answer yes. That's human nature. But the more you choose the healthy way, the more you'll feel the enduring pleasure of a better quality of life.

Chapter 22

Hope versus Fear

Summary

While it's easy to be consumed by fear, healing requires the constant re-kindling of hope.

What to Do

We've all had challenges in life. Recovering from concussion may be the greatest challenge you've faced. To keep going, you'll need to gain perspective on your emotions. When you fear all is lost, let yourself feel that feeling, but once you've processed it, focus on the reality that there's always the possibility of improvement.

As you're working on improving, know that it's okay to take breaks. Trying to do anything when you're mentally fatigued and cognitively challenged requires great effort. Deciding you need to coast for a day or a week is not giving up. Give yourself the option of resting intentionally, with a plan to return to the work of healing when ready.

In the recovery process, the key is to not give in to fear and slide into depression; one way to do that is by remembering that you can choose to be hopeful. Give yourself a pep talk. Know that there's a path of healing for you whether you've found it yet or not. Reach out to the people who love you. If you are spiritual, check in with that aspect of yourself. Do something you know will refresh your soul. Remember the challenges you have overcome in the past. Go forward.

Why

With concussion, so much focus is placed on the cognitive aspect that the emotional aspect can seem secondary. We seem to have the idea that our emotions are the passive result of how our lives are going. The reality is that without the right mindset, it's impossible to do the work needed to heal and we can influence that. Any injury that limits us can cause a deep sense of loss and lead to depression. To recover, we must acknowledge our feelings and strive to put hope before fear.

Our natural reaction to injury is to contract, both physically and emotionally. Muscles may tighten, the cranial system locks up and we withdraw into what feels safe. This closing down is a protective mechanism. It may serve a purpose initially, but over time it can create new problems. To heal we have to open back up.

Being hopeful is a way to look beyond your current situation to a better alternative. We don't always know what that alternative is, but hope can move us forward so that we're working towards recovery. Hope will get you out of bed in the morning (or afternoon). Hope will lead you to make good decisions. Hope will help you read the next page, take the supplements, do the exercise, make the appointment, and do it all again. Hope will transform you.

Personal Reflections

Personally, having hope versus succumbing to fear was my biggest challenge from my many concussions. I was so afraid that I would never recover. That being said, if it weren't for hope, I never would have made any recovery at all.

Every time I went to a doctor or read on the web that concussion treatment is about rest and a gradual return to activity, it was a hope killer. There was no path there, just waiting. By that point I'd already had plenty of rest and it hadn't worked for me.

I was fearful, but I didn't give up. I had hope so I tried different treatments. I had a pattern of almost recovering and then something would happen to set me back. Those setbacks became progressively worse each time.

But I was able to see that all was not lost. If I could improve for a short time, maybe there was something else I needed to do that would make those changes last. Hope kept me looking and learning.

Also, I think a lot of my perseverance was just obstinacy. I tend to be more intellectual than emotional, but I felt and hoped that since I had recovered to a point once, maybe I could do it again. Of course, there were also times when I wanted to just give up, quit my job, maybe quit my life. Thankfully, I have responsibilities in this world.

Some people like to say that everything happens for a reason. Fifteen or even five years ago if anyone had said that to me about all my concussions, I'm sure I would have said something very rude back. What possible reason could there be for all this suffering? However, I can see the good now. I am writing a book. I have made a web site to connect concussion patients and practitioners, (www.concussionprofessionals.com). I help others with PCS in my practice.

In all honesty, I'd much rather it had never happened. But it did. It happened to me, and it has happened to you. So, what good will come of it for you? Only hope will provide that answer. In the end you may appreciate certain things more. You will learn a lot about yourself. You will be stronger. Getting through this may be the biggest challenge you have faced. On the other side you will know your own strength.

Science and Specifics

Even on a physiological level, fear can prevent healing. Staying in a negative emotional state is stressful. When stressed, we release cortisol. Cortisol increases brain inflammation.

Conversely, hope is described as a cognitive process that leads to a mood rather than an emotion. Hope can be learned. Hope can be renewed through positive self-talk, inspirational reading, community, music, even humor and lightheartedness.

Some define hope as a way to maintain motivation toward achieving a goal. When it comes to concussion, the results on the path to recovery are hard to predict so the goals can be quite vague. But there is a path. As long as you can see that path and believe that you can go down it despite obstacles, you can hope for improvement. Any positive change in your condition will feed the hope you have for even more healing. Your goal needs to be staying on the path with the hope of some, however little, however slow, positive change.

Chapter 23

Anger

Summary

This chapter is for those who often feel irritated or are easily angered.

There is a type of reactive rage specific to head injury; it can be triggered by seemingly trivial annoyances or legitimate threats. Either way, it tends to be an overreaction. This can strain social relationships and be a source of shame, self-doubt, depression, even suicidal thoughts. On the other hand, recognizing the problem and working with it can provide a much-needed sense of pride and self-mastery.

What to Do

Physically, continue to work on reducing your brain inflammation with all of the strategies available to you. This alone can greatly reduce all types of emotional volatility. Do not consume caffeine; it will destabilize your nervous system's chemical environment. A more stable chemical environment means a more stable emotional state.

Also critical for emotional stability is having balance in neurotransmitters, especially dopamine and serotonin. Neurotransmitter balance can be affected by the stability of your blood sugar metabolism. For more on this subject, read the information on insulin resistance in Chapter 33: Regulating your Blood Sugar.

Dopamine and serotonin can also be influenced by nutraceuticals and pharmaceuticals. The supplement 5HTP supports serotonin production; if a short trial of 5HTP reduces anger, it would point to a lack of serotonin. St. John's Wort, SAMe, Tryptophan, and the B vitamins also support the serotonin pathway.

Before considering pharmaceutical intervention for your anger, consult a neuropsychologist. A neuropsychologist will be able to tell you and your neurologist or psychiatrist what related brain functions are involved with your emotional reactions, which will refine the choice of drug prescribed. [35]

Self-awareness is key for anger management. The problem is that self-awareness is weakened by head injury. Many head-injured people feel their expressions of anger are justified and appropriate. Having a head injury gives us plenty of reason to be angry. Even so, those reactions may be outsized in nature.

Awareness of having inappropriate fits of anger can be frightening and shameful. You may feel as if you are watching yourself, hearing what you are saying, but unable to stop. First you need to recognize that anger is fairly common among people with head injury. In that respect, it's normal. That doesn't mean that it's okay, but know that you're not the first person with a concussion to get angry. It's not really your fault.

Head-injury-related anger has been called defensive aggression. It happens in response to a perceived threat. [36] This threat could be what would otherwise be viewed as a minor irritant. If this happens to you, learn to recognize your triggers. These could be anything but tend to be situational. Miscommunication, changes in plans, physical discomfort, having to wait, having to rush, over-stimulation, confusion, other people's words or behavior, or difficulty doing things could be triggers for you. They can also be more physical or biochemical. Maybe you jarred your head a day or two ago, had a coffee or beer, ate too much sugar, went too long without a meal, slept poorly, or smelled a strong perfume or cleaning solution. When you are triggered, write down what did it. If you don't know what did it, describe the situation.

Building your knowledge of what triggers you will help you to deal with it the next time you feel it coming on. When it happens, ask yourself if what occurred really is a threat. The triggering event may be extremely irritating, a challenge to your concentration or comfort, but is it really a threat? This will help you diffuse the trigger enough to calm yourself.

Another way to calm yourself in the face of a triggering situation is to excuse yourself momentarily. Explaining why may worsen the situation; an excuse may be a better approach. If you do explain, do not blame or offend. Make it about you, not them. You need to own your own feelings if you want to change them. If you don't think you can talk without losing it, step away without saying a word. Then repeat the mantra: *let it go, let it go, let it go*. Once you've had a chance to settle down, congratulate yourself on successfully remaining composed and return if you think you can.

If it's too late and anger catches you by surprise, back away as soon as you realize what's happening. Again, you will need some techniques to calm yourself. This could be deep breathing, going for a walk, or positive self-talk. More often than not, an apology will be in order later. Let people know that you are sorry about your behavior, that it is neurological and that you are working on it.

If you need guidance in recognizing your triggers or developing calming techniques, there are anger management counselors and classes. Specifically for head trauma-related anger, there is a protocol called Anger Self-Management Training developed by Tessa Hart. This program has been shown to be significant and lasting in reducing anger for those with head injury. [37]

Cognitive Behavioral Therapy (CBT) is another approach. A therapist trained in CBT will help you recognize triggers and find ways to understand and manage your emotions.

Why

We need peace of mind. We need to keep our bonds of family and friendship intact. Bursts of anger, especially over seemingly trivial issues, can be very confusing to oneself and the people around you. The shame and embarrassment that typically follow won't help you heal. Driving people away may leave you feeling lonely and depressed.

On the other hand, becoming more self-aware, recognizing a problem, and taking steps to grow are small improvements that can boost confidence and provide a sense of accomplishment.

Personal Reflections

I've been on both sides of mTBI-associated defensive rage. My strongest memory of it is after a concussion that never should have happened. I let loose anger, emotion that had probably been festering for years, at the person responsible. As scary as it was to be totally out of control, it also felt good to finally be venting about a pattern I perceived in my life. My head injury-related lack of restraint has served me in other situations, particularly ones in which I otherwise would have swallowed my feelings. For the most part, however, my anger has been destructive. I cannot count the number of times I've apologized and I'm sure I haven't made my last apology.

When I work, as a practitioner, with other head-injured people, not everything always goes according to plan. No one health care provider has all the answers when it comes to post-concussion syndrome. Some of the treatment may be trial and error. Physical adjusting may be uncomfortable or cause a temporary flare-up. Progress may not happen with each treatment, or may be slower than expected. These can all trigger anger toward a provider. Please know that all of your practitioners are doing everything in their power to help you.

Science and Specifics

In dealing with brain trauma-associated anger, it helps to understand the nature of that anger and the cause.

Physiologically, certain areas of the frontal lobe of the brain and the connections to the limbic system may be injured or impaired due to inflammation. The frontal lobe is responsible for executive function, planning, adaptable thinking, self-control, and time management. The limbic system is associated with emotion.

You can see how problems in these areas could lead to irritability and anger. Per above, the particular type of anger experienced by those with TBI is defensive aggression; anger in reaction to a perceived threat. This is different from social or predatory aggression, which is more goal oriented. Research shows that in these aggressive reactions, there is an imbalance in dopamine and serotonin, with a surge in dopamine. [38] This chemical imbalance acts like a reflex that cannot be controlled even if we are aware that it's inappropriate.

Treatment for anger is available through a psychological training model or through pharmaceuticals. A study using Anger Self-Management Training (ASMT) had good results with 68% of the group reporting significant decreases in anger. In the study, the TBI patient had eight sessions with a therapist in which they learned self-monitoring and assessment and calming skills. Pharmaceuticals are aimed at restoring the dopamine-serotonin balance. These drugs are generally anti-depressants; but it doesn't mean that you've been diagnosed as depressed or are being treated for depression.

Caffeine alters neurotransmitter relationships in the brain in several ways that can contribute to anger (see Chapter 15). While it doesn't increase the amount of dopamine in the brain, it does increase the availability of dopamine receptors so there is more dopamine-related activity. [39] GABA, the neurotransmitter that buffers nerve activity, is decreased by caffeine, which also increases dopamine-related activity. [40] What's more, caffeine increases glutamate concentrations and can create neuroinflammation and neuro-excitotoxicity.

Chapter 24

Meditate

Summary

Before you can reconnect with the world, you need to reconnect with yourself.

What to Do

Make meditation part of your daily routine.

Why

Meditation is a way to quiet the mind. Not only does it give the overstimulated brain a chance to rest, it helps create a lasting sense of peace, relaxation, and awareness of oneself and one's surroundings.

Personal Reflections

In the earlier stages of my healing, I had a lot of head pain. This was not a typical headache-type pain, but felt like it was deeper in my head. It would move around from time to time. I would often notice it more when I was meditating and not getting other stimuli. They say the more you focus on something the bigger it gets, so rather than putting my attention on the pain, I would imagine my breath going right up into my head and my head widening with each inhale and narrowing with each exhale. The bones of the skull actually do this very subtly to pump fluid around the brain and spinal cord. I would imagine this fluid healing my poor aching brain and usually the pain would lessen. I imagine this kind of visualization might help pain anywhere in the body; you might want to give it a try.

Science and Specifics

There are many types of meditation. Many originate from philosophical or religious traditions, but that doesn't mean that you have to be a member of that tradition to use them. In modern times meditation has been kind of re-branded or classified as a form of mindfulness. Mindfulness is the idea of being self-aware in the present moment and acting with intention, two things often needing improvement when recovering from concussion.

The simplest form of meditation that I know and prefer comes from the Soto school of Zen Buddhism. They have a phrase, Shinkantaza, which translates to "just sit," and that is how you do it. Make yourself comfortable on a chair or cushion on the floor so you can keep good posture. Rest your hands on your lap. To cut out distractions, lower, but don't close your eyelids. Breath. From time to time, correct your posture. Keep sitting.

It's natural for thoughts to come up, just like it's natural for clouds to blow across the sky. Just treat your thoughts like clouds: acknowledge them, and then let them blow away. Over time, your mind should get less and less cloudy.

Some people like to follow their breath or count their breath. Others like to have a candle on the floor in front of them to watch. You can also do a meditative activity such as yoga, chi gung, or tai chi. These are a little busier and there is the distraction of trying to learn the activity, but they, too, can be very effective in developing mindfulness. A moving meditative activity may also help you improve your balance. On the other hand, if it's too challenging in terms of balance, it may be harder to enjoy the benefits of the calm, self-awareness of meditating. The key is to pick one or more ways, establish a routine, and stick to it.

One research study showed that mindfulness practices for mTBI patients, including meditation and yoga, resulted in consistent improvement of many symptoms. The most improvement was in depression and fatigue. Other areas of improvement were general mental health, physical health, cognitive performance, quality of life, and self-related processing (identifying one's own memories or personality traits). [41]

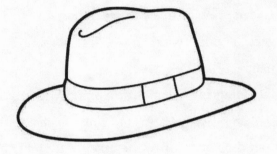

Part 5

Coping versus Working

Summary

The initial recommendation for all head injury is rest—not just resting the body, but resting the mind, as well. Like the body, the brain needs rest to heal. When the brain is ready, however, it needs exercise and work to recover. It's a matter of energy management.

Balancing out cognitive rest and cognitive work increases your brain's energy capacity. One way to achieve this balance is by figuring out how to cope effectively. In fact, coming up with coping strategies is an elegant way to leverage the rest/work relationship. Coping well allows the brain to rest. Generating the coping strategies is, in itself, a form of cognitive work.

The best coping strategy for brain fatigue is to simplify your life as much as possible and create a framework for your day-to-day routine. Having done that, you will have more energy to challenge specific neurological deficits through targeted therapies.

What to Do

First, identify a time of day when you're at your best; your mind is at its clearest, you have the least amount of distractions.

You are emotionally grounded. That's your time to work. Your first mental task is laying out your systems for coping.

Getting through the day provides many cognitive and emotional challenges. Identify your challenges. You may find it difficult to decide what to wear. Shopping or cooking may be overwhelming. Sleep may be an issue. Social situations may be challenging. Once you've identified what you need to work on, you can set up strategies around making it easier.

Pace yourself. Like every physical workout program, the key to long-term success is to challenge yourself enough to make progress without overexerting yourself. Therefore, the most critical skill you need to develop is self-awareness. This can be very difficult when you're feeling that your mind is not your own. Take a step back and try to observe yourself. This is a form of mindfulness and will serve you well. If you can recognize when your mind is starting to become fatigued and respect that, you'll greatly increase your chances of ongoing improvement.

When your mental stamina is running low, you will be best served by switching to an activity that requires less stamina or a different kind of focus. Do not try to push through when you are mentally fatigued, it will only create a hole that is harder to climb out of. An easy way to communicate the need for this to people around you, ones who understand your condition, is to tell them that you need a "brain break."

Why

Any activity that requires attention, cognition, or even emotional engagement can be considered work. When your brain is inflamed, your capacity for work is going to be low. Much of your cognitive energy may, in fact, be used in learning and implementing ways to lower your inflammation. Making lifestyle changes to lower and control that brain inflammation, and also using energy more efficiently, will add to your daily mental energy "bank."

Once your bank starts filling up, you will have more capacity for both daily activities and targeted brain recovery work. Targeted work means specific activities designed to improve areas of your brain that have deficits. This is the kind of work that promotes neuroplasticity, the ability to form new connections in your brain. Certain practitioners will direct you in these activities: neuropsychologists, functional neurologists, occupational therapists, speech pathologists, vestibular therapist, cognitive behavior therapist, neuro-optometrists and physical therapist that specialize in neurological recovery. Whew, that's a mouthful! I put neuropsychologist and functional neurologist at the beginning of the list, as they can help guide you to what approaches would be best for you. If you can't find such a provider near you, you may be able to be evaluated through tele-health. Best case scenario is finding a concussion clinic that can evaluate you, provide some services, and refer you to those they don't offer themselves.

Personal Reflections

Whenever my brain inflammation was activated, I found myself extremely fatigued. Fortunately for me, as a chiropractor, my office comes with several treatment tables. I got very good at scheduling several patients close together with naps between groups. In retrospect, it would have been much better for me to have just taken a month off, but those breaks were a coping mechanism that helped me get through the tougher times and slowly build back my capacity for mental energy.

Science and Specifics

In every cell of your body are specialized organelles called mitochondria. These mitochondria produce ATP (Adenosine tri-Phosphate), the fuel for that cell. Concussion puts a huge energy demand on the brain. At the same time the neuroinflammatory process can damage the mitochondria. Together that causes brain fatigue and limits the brain's ability to heal.

To become stable, you must give the mitochondria a good working environment by reducing neuroinflammation. To recover you must use your energy wisely so as not to overwork your mitochondria. On the other hand, a cell will produce more mitochondria if it's challenged. This is the basis of the rest/work relationship.

Chapter 25

Sleep

Summary

The most important part of managing your physical and mental energy is starting with as much of both as possible. There is no replacement for a good night's sleep. Consistent sleep is essential for concussion recovery, but many people have problems with their quality of sleep after concussion. Brain inflammation affects your amount and quality of sleep, and poor sleep will increase brain inflammation. So, the issue must be approached from both sides.

What to Do

For the head injured, the first step in getting a good night's sleep is controlling brain inflammation. Please read Part 3: Brain Inflammation, First Steps and Part 6: What the Brain Needs to Heal. Pay particular attention to Chapter 32: Regulate your Blood Sugar. Sugar dys-regulation is a major cause of sleep disturbance.

Stress contributes to sleep problems. If you have been concussed, you are stressed, end of story. We are very complex beings and how you deal with stress is a personal matter. It would be an oversimplification and an insult to say that any one problem you may be having could be solved by stress reduction, alone. We do know that it helps and that we must find our own ways to do that.

PTSD, Post-Traumatic Stress Disorder may also be a factor in sleep disturbance. For this you will need psychological help. EMDR, Eye Movement Desensitization and Reprocessing, is one therapy that has proved to be very effective in resolving PTSD related to specific events.

No matter what the root cause of your sleep disturbance, make sure to listen to your body and brain. If you feel like you need sleep, you do. It's fine to nap, though you don't want to sleep so long during the day that you can't sleep at night. It's also fine to go to bed early. You may want to have longer regular sleep hours both during the day and at night. Conversely, if you have trouble staying asleep, you may need to shorten your hours of sleep so you are more tired when you go to bed. Six hours of solid sleep may be more restful than ten hours of frequently interrupted sleep. The key is to listen to your body.

You may need to change your lifestyle to promote sleep. Practice what's called sleep hygiene. This is planning around sleep and taking steps to make it easier to fall asleep and stay asleep. Here are some suggestions:

- Have a regular sleep schedule
- Have a regular routine for preparing to sleep
- Write down all the things you'd like to do the next day and leave your list away from the bedroom so you don't need to think about them in bed
- If you are not light sensitive, increase exposure to natural sunlight or other bright light during the day
- Exercise during daylight hours
- Begin dimming lights at least an hour before bed
- Do not watch TV or use screens an hour before bed
- Change your settings on your screens to nighttime (low blue light) if you are light sensitive and leave them that way all the time. If you're not light sensitive, set them so the night setting comes on when it's getting dark out.
- Put your Wi-Fi on a timer so it goes off at least one hour before bed

- Only use your bedroom for sleep, changing clothes, and intimacy

- Keep the temperature of your room below 70 degrees F, 20 degrees C

- Do not sleep in other rooms of the house

- Do some gentle stretches, meditate, or pray before going to sleep

- Eat at regular times and do not eat before bed

- If you do snack, make it protein (nuts, cheese, or a hard-boiled egg are good options), rather than a sugar-or carbohydrate-based snack

- Reduce or eliminate caffeine consumption

- Eliminate alcohol consumption

- Limit liquids before bed

There are medications and supplements for sleep; the issue with these is that you can become dependent. The hormone melatonin is available as a supplement. It improved sleep disturbance in 67% of sleep disturbed concussion patients. [42] However, taking melatonin can reduce your own production, dysregulate your system, and cause you to need more of the supplement for the same effect. Melatonin isn't a good long-term solution, but it can help as a short-term reset of circadian rhythms. Acupuncture can also be helpful with insomnia.

In the long run, you must solve the root problem of your sleep disturbance. Reduce brain inflammation, have healthy sugar regulation, manage stress, and address psychological trauma. Then you will be on your way to more rest and recovery.

Why

A correlation has been found between a decreased level of consciousness post-injury and an increase in sleep disturbance. [43] A correlation has also been found between sleep issues and both the next day[44] and prolonged symptoms. [45] During sleep the body, including the brain, heals. Learning and memory, two functions greatly affected by concussion and needed for recovery, are consolidated during the REM or dreaming cycle of sleep.

Personal Reflections

After my injuries, it seems all I could do was sleep. At that time, I was a member of a networking group that met at 7 a.m. every Tuesday. This meant I had to wake up an hour before I usually did once a week. Even before my concussions, this change in my routine would throw me off for a day or two. After my initial concussions, it was completely unmanageable, and I had to take a medical leave of absence from the group.

That helped but did not solve the problem of being tired all the time. Chiropractic offices come with tables that are meant to be laid on. Your employer might not be so accommodating. I was very happy to have a place to lie down between patients and I was able to maintain some income, but long-term, I would've been better served by giving myself a leave of absence from my work, or if I'd been employed by someone else, filing for temporary disability.

This speaks to the need to seriously rest after initial injury. The brain inflammation-sleep disturbance cycle needs to be broken as soon as possible.

Science and Specifics

Studies report that people tend to sleep more in the first month after a concussion, but then have difficulty sleeping after that. However, post-concussion sleep patterns vary from person to person. [46] Some continue to sleep a lot, others find it difficult to fall asleep, while others awaken often or early and have trouble returning to sleep.

The sleep cycle is part of our daily circadian rhythm, which also includes the body's hormonal rhythm and eating and digesting cycles. It's regulated by an area of the brain that is directly stimulated by light. That's why much of sleep hygiene is related to experiencing the natural cycle of light and dark.

Inflammation

Research has shown that brain inflammation contributes to sleep disturbance. In one series of experiments, rats that had been modified so they could not activate inflammatory microglial cells of the brain were given concussions. These rats did not have as much sleep interruptions at night compared to normal rats with concussion. [47] Other studies have shown that sleep deprivation causes brain inflammation through microglial activation, [48] so what we have here is a vicious cycle. Brain inflammation causes sleep issues and lack of sleep causes brain inflammation.

In one experiment, rats treated with Resolvin E1, which is derived from the essential fatty acid EPA, had decreased microglial activation and improved sleep. [49] Another study showed that taking Aspirin with EPA increased levels of RvE1 production. [50]

Chapter 26

Routine is your Friend

Summary

Struggling with how to do something simple can be very frustrating. We have many daily or weekly tasks. Before head injury, we didn't have to think about these things, they were automatic. When you have a head injury, multi-step tasks and planning are typically a challenge. They can tax our mental energy and become a source of great frustration. The simplest way to deal with these tasks is to establish routines that, over time, turn into automatic habits.

What to Do

Start each day with the same plan, a list of routine tasks. For every task, break it down into smaller steps. It doesn't matter how simple the step is, include it and put the steps in order. For example:

Take a shower:

1. Take off pajamas
2. Turn on water
3. Adjust temperature
4. Get in shower
5. Wash head to toe, shampoo hair, wash face, wash body
6. Turn off water
7. Dry off

Do this for as many tasks as needed.

Arrange items in the order you might use them. Keep your belts near you pants in the closet. Socks near the shoes. Bacon near the eggs.

A pill organizer for supplements, with separate sections labeled with the day and morning, noon and night, is very helpful. Filling it once a week makes things much easier than having to remember what to take each day. For liquid supplements, put something in the organizer such as a bean or marble, corresponding with the time you need to take them, as a reminder.

Create a place for everything so you don't need to run around looking for things. For instance, put a tray by the door or on your dresser where you empty your pockets. Have a hook where you hang your purse or keys. If you're constantly losing your glasses or your phone, make an effort to put them in the same spot every time you're done using them, even if you have to walk through the house to do it. You will save yourself a lot of effort later.

Pick a spot where you can put items you need to take back and forth to work or school — this might be a bag that you hang up in the same place every evening. Put items in that place/bag the night before, when you're thinking about taking them. This is much easier than trying to remember everything right before leaving. If you're at work and remember that you need something from home, write it on a note and put it in the bag or stick it on your wallet or phone. When you get home replace the note with the item.

Set up triggers at the end of one task that will remind you what other tasks need to be done. For example, I keep my deodorant next to my shaver in the medicine cabinet. When I put the deodorant back, I take out the shaver and put it on the vanity to remind me I need to use it after I get dressed. The same could be done for a makeup bag or lotion.

Write down routines or print them out. Post them where you'll be doing the activity so you can refer to them. (Laminate the one for the shower!) As you repeat the activity over time, you will need the list less. It will seem like a small victory, but recovery is about small victories.

Once you have lists for the minor daily and weekly tasks in order, you'll need a system for planning the unique activities of any given day or week. That system can be a routine, too. You may want to list out everything you'd like to do. I use Stephen Covey's Time Management Matrix, which divides tasks into four squares. Take a sheet of paper and write "Urgent" and "Not Urgent" above the top two squares. Then write "Important" on the left side next to the upper square and "Not Important" on the left side, next to the lower square. I take my list and put each item into one of the four quadrants. Items that fall into the Important/Urgent category usually take priority and the ones in the Not Important/Not Urgent almost never get done, but that's ok. Another system recommends doing items that will take very little time first just so they are done and not hanging over your head. I set up my squares every Monday morning, number my top three priority tasks, and forget about the rest until I've done what I can on those.

For larger tasks, divide them into steps and cross them off as you do them. Major projects should also be broken down and the steps added to a calendar. What's nice about a calendar app is you can set repeating events and schedule individual steps of projects. You can also move items around easily. If you get a reminder to do something and you are behind, no big deal.

If you're your sharpest at a certain time of day, use that time to plan. Set up your routines, plan for that day or, if you're best in the evening, plan for the next day. Lay out your clothes, your meal plan, and the ingredients needed. Check in with your goals for the day or week and make any needed changes. Have specific times that you make phone calls or write emails. Silence devices at other times. As all these routines become habits, you won't need to think about them.

Whatever system you create, make it part of your routine. It will help bring order to your life, lessen the cognitive load on your brain, and renew your sense of competence.

Personal Reflections

I included this chapter because there were times when I would wake up in the morning, go into the bathroom and not know what to do. I'm sure there were plenty of times I washed my hair twice because I couldn't remember if I'd done it or not. That's when I started putting together daily routines and breaking them down into steps.

There is no shame in being injured, but I know that there were times that I felt shame or embarrassment for myself because I had difficulty doing simple things. This would easily turn into despair or fear that I would never get better or be the person I was. Here I was, a guy who put himself through college, became a Doctor of Chiropractic, started my own business and I couldn't take a shower.

It's not just about getting through the day. It's not just about having more mental energy to do other things. It is about regaining control of your life. It's about knowing that you can recover. If you can re-learn how to take a shower or make your breakfast, you can relearn how to organize a meeting, fix a car, and write a computer program. You may not be able to do it right away or as well as you used to, and it may take more time, but you can do it. Just keep trying and use these strategies to make it easier for yourself.

Science and Specifics

A lot is involved in learning or doing even a simple task. Both involve cognition and memory. Different kinds of cognition and memory connect to different (and related) parts of the brain. Considering there's so much variation in what areas of the brain are affected from one concussion to the next, it's not surprising which brain functions are affected varies greatly from one person to the next.

Research related to the different functions involved with planning and doing a task and the different types of memory involved in mTBI populations is inconsistent. Procedural memory is a form of long-term memory that allows us to do routine tasks without consciously thinking about them. Like riding a bike. Some studies say procedural memories we've already made are not affected much by mTBI. [51]Though it does take longer for someone who's been concussed to form new procedural memories.

Complex tasks that require more planning or being broken into steps (and remembering those steps) are more challenging for the mTBI patient. We also have a harder time remembering to do things we planned to do whether we made that plan five minutes ago or a week ago. [52]

The strategies I've outlined in this chapter are coping mechanisms. I don't like that term because it implies that you're stuck with a condition forever and have to find workarounds. There may be areas of your brain that have permanent damage; however, we are resilient. Our brains can form new connections. We can re-learn old skills and learn new ones. Our memory can improve. We can become more organized. These are tools to make your life simpler and easier, less taxing on your fatigued brain. Over time, these same tools can allow for recovery and healing.

Chapter 27

Clutter

Summary

Lessening clutter in your life reduces mental clutter and brain fatigue.

What to Do

Minimize sensory distractions.

Tidy up! Organize your stuff and put it away. Get rid of things you don't need. Store what you rarely use.

Create a peaceful environment for yourself.

Why

A messy home or workplace provides infinite distraction. Every time you sense something, your brain gives it a tiny bit of attention. Ordinarily a slight, unconscious distraction would have little meaning, but for the tired, inflamed brain, these little distractions tax our limited capacity. This applies to visual, auditory, and even olfactory sensations.

It's much easier to find something if you don't have to remember where you put it. If you are organized and put things back where you typically keep them, you'll spend much less time looking for things.

The fewer things you have, the easier they are to manage. It's much easier to decide which pair of shoes to wear if you keep the three pairs you wear the most upfront in your closet. You don't have to throw the rest away, but you might want to put them in the back of the closet or on a high shelf, where you don't have to see them whenever you're getting ready to leave home.

Personal Reflections

In college, a good friend of mine once asked me how much clearer my mind would be if I didn't have to think about stepping over a dirty sock on the floor every time I walked through a room. I think he was just annoyed that I was messy, but I've thought a lot about that since, and he was right. Minor distractions add up. Thank you, Eric.

Abraham Lincoln is quoted as saying, "If I only had an hour to cut down a tree, I would spend the first 45 minutes sharpening my ax." You can apply this phrase to many things. I think of it most when I decide to focus on one task and have the stuff from five other tasks and random notes all over my desk. For me, the ax-sharpening is cleaning my desk.

I tend to keep some order within the chaos, so it may be just a matter of grouping related items into folders, but if the desk is too busy, I have another desk. The other desk has nothing on it, ever. I can take something from the messy desk to the clean desk and put all my focus on it. When I'm done, I take it back to the messy desk or put it away. I love my clean desk.

The same applies in the kitchen. When I want to prepare a meal, I must start with a clean kitchen. That means; put away any clean dishes and clean any dirty dishes first. My wife must think I'm very tidy. The truth is I can't handle the distraction. I secretly wonder if she knows this...

Science and Specifics

Neurologically, it has been shown using functional MRI that attention is competitive. On the simplest level that means if you're trying to concentrate on one thing, anything else in your perception will pull your attention away from what you're trying to focus on. [53] This is especially true for the head-injured, who have difficulty filtering out meaningless sensory stimulus. This demonstrates how much cognitive bandwidth can be saved for the concussed just by being tidy.

Chapter 28

Fake It 'til you Make It

Summary

As a head-injured person, certain situations can be overwhelming and feel like work. We may want to avoid those feelings and the associated energy drain, but that would mean missing out. Plus it's important to exercise your brain. One option is to behave "as if" we can meet that specific cognitive, social, or emotional challenge as a form of practice in controlled situations. Doing so may help you relearn or become more comfortable in those scenarios.

What to Do

Identify a cognitive, emotional or social challenge you currently have. Consciously prepare strategies to either cope with or present yourself as not having them. Put yourself in the situation that brings up the challenge. Use your strategies or act "as if" you did not have the challenge. Have an exit strategy to use before the situation is too challenging.

For example:

You have a hard time reading. Maybe you jumble the words in a sentence. You read a sentence, but it has no meaning to you. Your eyes don't track well on the page. Choose a short passage to read. Read one paragraph out loud. As you read, take brief notes on the key points or events. Read the next paragraph and do the same. Before you become mentally fatigued, stop. Read over your notes. Do they make sense? Do you comprehend what you just read? If so, congratulations. If not, come back to the same passage later. Read your notes on the first paragraph, then read the paragraph out loud. Clarify your notes. Proceed until finished. Re-read your notes. Do this until you can congratulate yourself.

Perhaps you are dis-inhibited in conversation. You say things that might not be appropriate, relevant or even what you truly think. Perhaps your timing is off. You think of something to say after the conversation has moved on. If you are going into a social situation, think of some neutral topics that might come up.

Think of something brief and true to yourself that you might say about a particular topic. If the topic comes up, or you bring it up yourself, say your one thing. Then let the others move forward with it. Otherwise simply nod and say, "I see" or "uh huh," neither of which mean you agree, just that you are listening. Ask questions. People feel connected to people who are interested in their opinion. If someone asks you a question you're not ready to respond to, say you're not sure or would need to think about it. Then ask them what they think. When you need to leave or take a break, do it. Have an out; a reason you may have to leave early or take a break. Congratulate yourself on a successful social interaction.

Why

There is a difference between symptoms and personality. After their injury, many people suffer from a whole range cognitive issues and emotional challenges: social anxiety, irritability, anger, depression, feelings of overwhelm, general anxiety, mood swings, or lack of emotion. When symptoms go on for a long time, you may feel as if your personality has changed. Others may feel this way too. Certainly, in the moment, the way your personality presents may be altered, but if it weren't for the symptoms, you might be your "usual self." Sometimes we can lose track of that usual self and it may take some work to bring it back to the surface.

This in part is the realm of Cognitive Behavioral Therapy (CBT). CBT helps you become more aware of your deficits and the triggers that bring them out. Once you've developed your awareness, you can make a conscious plan for what to do in those situations. If you practice this, like anything else, it will become easier and more natural.

As you work to address the root cause of symptoms, there will be less of a need to act "as if," but the effort you put in before then will lay the groundwork for reclaiming old ways or even creating better new ways. There are certain situations where the root cause may be difficult to resolve. In these cases, your work to self-regulate will have to serve as an ongoing adaptation, an accomplishment you can be proud of.

Personal Reflections

I've never been much of a social person; I'm the guy who has a few close friends. I can say anything to these friends and they continue to accept me. My initial head injuries came three years after moving to a new location where I knew my brother, his wife, and I met my own wife. Otherwise, I didn't have close people in the area. My injury took me out of the martial arts circle of acquaintances and friends I saw at class and left me with no social activities. They also left me without the energy to seek out new social groups for quite a while.

When my child started kindergarten, I was so pleased because I thought it would be a great opportunity to be part of a community. The problem was that I was a little too excited. The first five-year-old's birthday party we went to, I spoke to the people there as if they were good friends. I brought up a politically charged topic about which I really should have kept my mouth shut. I assumed everyone would agree with me, but one person strongly disagreed, and I just kept talking and digging myself a deeper hole. Sadly, this person was well connected socially and my "openness" on the topic pretty much put an end to the opportunity of making new friends.

This was the first time I became aware of how much my concussions had impacted my ability to read social situations and how little control I had over expressing my opinions. It was a real wakeup call for me. Since then, I try to use the strategy I outlined above when going into new social situations. It doesn't mean I don't express myself; it just means that I'm more cautious and wait till I've built a firm relationship to speak with the openness I'd use with a good friend. I've gotten better at it.

Science and Specifics

The brain is amazing at adapting; it's called plasticity. Plasticity is when the brain re-wires itself and creates new connections; it's how we learn, and how we recover skills we've lost due to brain injury. Many cognitive, emotional, and social skills can be learned or re-learned through intention and practice.

The multiple factors involved in brain injury may make plasticity more challenging: neuroinflammation, hormonal or neurotransmitter changes, or actual brain damage. But that does not mean it's not possible.

Every small accomplishment you make bring you closer to making yourself whole. This is true for head-injured and non-head injured people alike. A strategy that you use as an adaptation today may become unnecessary tomorrow. What you need to remember is that even the ongoing use of an adaptation is an accomplishment. Recognizing that, alone, will change your brain chemistry, making progress in all areas more possible.

Chapter 29

Music Nature Pets and Love

Summary

Gratitude, awe, and love can provide us with a respite from physical and emotional challenges. This respite serves as an inner sanctuary to which we can retreat, a place to regenerate our state of being. Certain environments, beings, or activities can help us reach and enjoy this state.

What to Do

Retreating to our inner sanctuary is not so much about doing anything but *being* in a particular way. The simplest description is being in a state of love, just not with a person. Each of us appreciates particular things; it may be music, good food, nature, art, or an animal. Certain open-ended activities, such as knitting, swimming, gardening, crafts, even cleaning the house may give you a sense of joy. The idea is to be in a softly focused state of mind, experiencing feelings of gratitude, pleasure, and even awe, without the demand of conscious thought or completing a goal. This is a little vacation for the mind.

Why

Feeling grateful for—and lost in awe at—a certain activity overlaps with gratitude and awe in being alive. Depending on how you were injured, you may be lucky to be alive. While I know it's hard to think this way, you are lucky to be as well as you are. It could have been worse. If you weren't taking the steps you are now, it may have gotten worse. If you've made any progress in recovery, then it really was worse. When we get outside ourselves and really appreciate something, we can do that because we have a relationship with it. That relationship is unspoken, and free of judgment, expectations, or demands. As part of that relationship, in that moment you are also in a state of unconditional love for yourself; unspoken, free of judgment, expectations or demands.

Personal Reflections

Like many ideas expressed in this book, this one came to me accidentally or in hindsight. I have my dog, my garden, and all the open spaces around my home to thank for the peace of mind they have given me on so many occasions. I honestly believe that my dog has saved my life many times. Of course, I am lucky to have the best dog in the world, just like you, if you have a dog.

Science and Specifics

I could not find any scientific studies on the benefits for concussed people of being in a state of gratitude, awe, or love. I do think we all know it's a good idea. The same goes for being with pets or doing hobbies.

Plenty of studies reveal how being in nature reduces stress. [54] And we know stress can create or worsen brain inflammation. That is enough evidence for me.

As a head-injured person, if you think about your state of mind or what kind of mood you are generally in, you might say confused, tired, angry, irritated, depressed or out of control. None of these are positive. The beauty of being in a state of gratitude, awe, or love, is that it requires no thought, and no matter how tired or how much pain you may be in, it takes you out of all those other negative states.

You may be wondering why I don't suggest experiencing love with a significant other, friend, or family member. Of course, it's nice and it's healing to love and be loved. We need this kind of love as well. The trouble with people is that we tend to have expectations of one another. If one feels they are not having their expectations met or meeting the other's expectations, it creates a certain tension. Dogs and trees do not have expectations and we don't expect much from them. Just being is what we are going for.

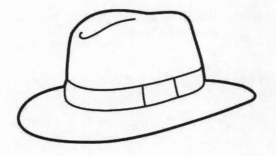

Part 6

What the Brain Needs to Heal

Summary

The healing brain's needs are simple. How they are met is complicated. In the next few chapters, those needs will be broken down and simplified as much as possible.

What to Do

Give your brain the opportunity to heal by providing:

- Fuel
  - Oxygen
  - Glucose or Ketones
- A controlled, balanced environment
- Raw materials
- Stimulus

Why

The entire body has an amazing capacity to heal. The brain needs the same fundamentals as the rest of the body, but the brain's unique and complicated function makes providing those fundamental needs more complex. Nevertheless, given the opportunity, the brain is capable of great healing.

Personal Reflections

There are two real tragedies in the field of concussion treatment. The first is the Rest and Return model. This is the idea that all concussions will get better all by themselves with rest. If you are reading this book, you know that is wrong.

The second tragedy is treating the brain through stimulus before the other basic needs have been met. You cannot rebuild a house that is still on fire. There are many very powerful, valid means of rehabilitating specific areas of the brain by exercising them, but to do so before there is fuel, a balanced controlled environment, and raw materials is, in my opinion, a waste of time and could even prolong suffering.

A lot of healing will take place from stimulus we encounter in our daily lives once the brain is able to produce fuel, has a stable low inflammation environment, and the raw materials it needs. If more targeted brain rehabilitation is needed, the progress will be much faster and lasting once basic needs are met.

Science and Specifics

All cells produce fuel using oxygen and either fat, glucose or ketones. Brain cells cannot use fat. The fuel is produced via structures inside each cell called mitochondria. Concussion can harm mitochondria in brain cells. Oxygen and glucose regulation can also be impacted by traumatic brain injury.

This damage and dysregulation are mostly due to the inflammatory environment of the injured brain. Restoring energy production means controlling inflammation first. To do that the brain needs a stable, well-regulated environment.

The Blood Brain Barrier (BBB) is a filter. It selectively allows chemicals in and out of the brain. When concussed, this filter can become leaky, which disrupts the brain's environment and causes more inflammation. To heal the brain, the BBB must also heal.

The raw materials needed to heal the BBB and brain have an effect on chemical reactions that cause inflammation. The raw materials can also become part of the neurons themselves. For example, DHA is an essential fatty acid that both affects chemical reactions and becomes part of the neurons. Many other supplements may be needed depending on the degree of inflammation.

Finally, the brain needs the right kind of stimulus at the right time and in the right amount balanced with needed rest. This can be very injury specific.

Chapter 30

Oxygen

Summary

The brain needs oxygen to function and even more to heal. Traumatic brain injury can limit blood flow to the brain. It's very important to address the causes of those limits and remedy them.

Symptoms of poor brain circulation may include:

- Dizziness when standing or sitting up quickly
- Brain gets tired easily
- Poor focus
- Can't think without caffeine or exercise

- Cold hands, feet or nose

- Poor nail health or fungal growth on toes

- White nail beds instead of pink

What to Do

Consult your medical doctor or functional medicine practitioner to rule out anemia, (weak blood). Consult a cardiologist regarding your heart health.

Exercise within your tolerance range (see Chapter 31).

Do not smoke anything.

Consider taking supplements that may lower blood pressure.[*] These are:

Riboflavin (B2)

Magnesium

Ginkgo biloba

Vinpocetine

Adenosine

N-Acetyl L-Carnitine

Alpha-GPC

Huperzine A

---

[*] Statements regarding supplements have not been evaluated by the FDA. Supplements are not intended to diagnose, treat, cure or prevent disease.

Hawthorn

Consider Hyperbaric Oxygen Therapy (HBOT).

Why

Every cell needs oxygen to produce energy. The brain needs a lot of energy, so it's a major consumer of oxygen. Even though the brain is about 2% of our body weight, it uses about 20% of the oxygen we consume. [55] The injured brain needs even more oxygen to heal because it needs more energy.

Just when the brain needs more oxygen, it may be harder to get if blood flow is reduced by blood vessel damage or pressure caused by inflammation. Without enough oxygen, healthy neurons cannot function. They may become damaged. Damaged neurons may die and cause more loss of function and inflammation.

Personal Reflections

Oxygen is something we generally don't think about. We just breath as much as we need and that's the end of the story. It never occurred to me that my injured brain would benefit from more oxygen. Fortunately for me an acupuncturist recommended I start exercising a little in the morning. At that time, I was always fatigued and fairly depressed. The idea of exercising wasn't appealing, but if it got me out of that funk, I'd do it. Even then I didn't make the exercise/oxygen/brain health connection; I figured it was all about hormones, energy production, and the blood circulation clearing out toxins and refreshing tissues in the whole body. I learned that I felt better when I exercised, but I didn't realize that oxygen was part of it. You can learn more about the benefit of exercise in the next chapter.

A lot of head-injured people become depressed. Exercise requires motivation that may just not be there for some. Many people may be physically unable to exercise. There are times when it's not good to exercise, such as the first two weeks after injury or after a re-injury. But oxygen is still important during those periods. Fortunately, we have the more passive ways of increasing oxygen to the brain, including supplements and Hyperbaric Oxygen Therapy (HBOT).

My impression is that the supplements are helpful, but much more helpful in conjunction with exercise. HBOT can be very helpful, but can be expensive. Insurance doesn't recognize HBOT as a treatment for post-concussion syndrome (PCS). Maybe someday. If it's difficult to find a facility offering HBOT therapy near you, it may be better to buy or rent an HBOT chamber for yourself.

Science and Specifics

Using SPECT imaging, twelve out of twenty patients with minor head injury showed less brain blood flow in areas of low function. [56] Some severe head injury patients initially have either low or high blood pressure (BP). Low BP right after injury is associated with less recovery. It's not clear if high BP right after injury is damaging or not, but ongoing high BP can be a sign of poor autonomic nervous system function and overactive adrenal glands. High blood pressure can damage the blood brain barrier. It can also cause swelling in the brain, which increases pressure in the skull and ultimately decreases blood flow. [57]

Regular exercise increases the amount of oxygen the blood can carry. It also stimulates the growth of new blood vessels. After just five minutes of intense exercise, the body produces a chemical called endothelial Nitric Oxide, (eNOS). This chemical relaxes blood vessels, decreasing BP and increasing blood flow. The supplements listed above in "What to Do" work to increase oxygenation to the brain either by supporting eNOS production or lowering BP. It's most effective to take them about thirty minutes before exercise.

HBOT

Hyperbaric Oxygen Therapy (HBOT) involves being in a sealed chamber or room in which the oxygen concentration and air pressure is higher than normal. This pushes more oxygen into the blood. Oxygen is normally carried by red blood cells (RBC). HBOT provides oxygen to meet the carrying capacity of RBC, plus it dissolves oxygen into the liquid blood plasma. This provides more oxygen for the healing brain. The dissolved oxygen can also travel through damaged blood vessels that RBC cannot and reach areas that would not get oxygen otherwise.

While there is some disagreement in the scientific community about whether HBOT is effective for treating PCS, some studies have shown good results in both cognitive abilities and quality of life measurements. These results are thought to come from increased nerve repair, stimulation of new blood vessel growth, stimulation of new nerve connections (neuroplasticity), and even stimulation of new nerve formation from stem cells in the brain. These results were seen in PCS patients after forty HBOT sessions over two months even when done one to five years after they were injured. [58]

Chapter 31

Exercise

Summary

Certain types of exercise in limited amounts can help the brain heal.

What to Do

During the first two weeks after a concussion or re-injury, rest. Low-intensity, low-impact exercise is okay, but avoid medium- or high-intensity exercise. That would be exercise that increases your heartrate to 50-85% of your maximum heartrate.

Maximum heartrate is generally 220 beats per minute minus your age. It's easier to judge by how you are breathing. Medium intensity means that you could talk, but not sing. High intensity means it's hard to talk.

It's generally safe to start exercising two weeks after your injury. Begin with just a few minutes of medium-intensity, low-impact exercises and see how you feel in two days. (There are added benefits if the exercise is done first thing in the morning.) If you don't have a negative reaction, work up to five to ten minutes a day at higher intensity low impact. Then repeat two or three times a day.

If you do have a negative reaction, either right away or within two days, it could either be from inflammation or the type of exercise you're doing is aggravating an injured part of your brain. This could be a direct chemical or physical aggravation or an aggravation from demanding too much focus, co-ordination, or balance.

Why

Compared to resting, exercise within the first week or so of injury increases brain inflammation. By two weeks post-injury, intense exercise decreases brain inflammation. [59]I recommend intense yet low-impact, such as fast walking, swimming, cycling, or using an elliptical trainer, because it doesn't shock your brain with jarring motions. I would also avoid resistance training or weightlifting. These increase internal pressure when straining and may give you a headache or flare you up.

Regular exercise increases the oxygen-carrying capacity of red blood cells. If done within fifteen minutes of waking up, it changes the pattern of morning cortisol release so you will not wake up as tired and will have more motivation.

Intense exercise reduces inflammation and helps the brain recover. Just five minutes of intense exercise has been shown to raise the level of chemicals in the brain that:

- Repair and build blood vessels
- Build links between neurons
- Increase nerve development in the memory center
- Regulate the immune response in the body and brain
- Improve mood
- Decrease pain
- Reduce microglial priming
- Shift primed microglial cells from the M1 to M2 expression
- Improve motivation[60]
- Lower insulin resistance[61]

Personal Reflections

My first concussion happened in an aikido class. Aikido is a martial art that uses a lot of pivoting, pinning, and throwing the opponent by spinning them one way or another. After my injury, as I thought I was recovering, I would test myself by seeing if I could go back to aikido. Every time I tried, I would walk away with a raging headache and a relapse of symptoms that would last a week or more. I thought it was the jarring motions to the brain. I'm sure that was part of it, but now I understand that it was also the type of movement. My brain areas that monitor balance and the sense of where the body is in space (the cerebellum and vestibular system), were being overwhelmed.

Based on my failures at returning to aikido, I stayed away from exercise in general until an acupuncturist told me that I might have less fatigue if I did a little aerobic exercise first thing in the day. I started riding my bike to work, which was just five minutes away, downhill. That really helped me turn a corner in my recovery and showed me the benefit of exercise for the brain.

Soon after, I started swimming regularly. I love swimming for head injury because it is completely non-impact. There is a meditative aspect to it for me. The movement is a cross crawl which helps the two sides of the brain connect and talk to each other. Also, I have always been a weak swimmer. I get tired and winded quickly so it's the perfect high intensity exercise for me. At my best, I can only swim for five to ten minutes.

Since I couldn't do aikido, I opted to do tai chi. That also challenges our sense of balance, but it's very slow and no one throws you on the floor. While I didn't know it at the time, I see now that tai chi was very helpful in rehabbing the balance areas of my brain. Over the years, I've wondered if I could go back to aikido. At this point I think I might be able to handle it, though it would be a risk. At my current age, the prospect of being thrown on the floor is not appealing. I never was very good at rolling.

I must say that, as much as I personally hate exercise, it has been a major key to my recovery. I am quite sure that if I'd changed the type of exercise I was trying earlier on, my recovery would've been much quicker and more complete. If I'd known how little was needed to make a big change, I'm sure I would have started earlier.

One beautiful thing about exercise is that it's all you. It's an action you can take for yourself to heal yourself. If you have ever felt helpless in the face of your injuries, exercise is your opportunity to take charge. Releasing all those chemicals and getting that oxygen to your brain will not just heal it physically; the accomplishment of doing it yourself will help heal you emotionally and spiritually.

Science and Specifics

Exercise is important for recovery, but you have to be careful with it, especially right after an injury or when you have a lot of primed microglial cells. Exercise creates free radicals and oxidative stress, which causes inflammation and increases the M1 expression of primed microglial cells. At the same time, during exercise, the muscles release a lot of anti-inflammatory chemicals to counter-act inflammation and shift the microglial cells into the M2 state. The anti-inflammatory benefits can last for hours, but if your system is very sensitive, the initial rush of free radicals may trigger an inflammatory response that can spiral out of control. If the microglial cells react, you can get more activation or priming. Symptoms may come a day or two after this added inflammation.

You need to start slowly. Find that sweet spot in time and intensity that gives you the benefits of the exercise without a negative reaction. As your system becomes less inflamed and reactive, you will be able to increase. The good news for those of us who don't enjoy exercising is that you only need five to ten minutes of intense exercise to get the maximum benefit. The bad news for people who really enjoy exercising for long periods at high intensity is that, if they're brain injured, it may not be the best thing to do for their brain for quite some time.

In addition to the inflammatory response, you may have a negative reaction if it's too challenging to an injured part of your brain. This could be from the type of exercise you are doing or from the environment you are in when you do it. Exercise that requires a lot of concentration and focus, such as doing core exercises or working out with a Bosu ball, may tax the brain. The same goes for activities that require reacting with hand-eye coordination, such as tennis. Up and down and turning motions can also challenge the balance system. Stairmaster and treadmill exercise in which your body thinks it should be moving in relation to your surroundings, but isn't, can confuse and tire the cerebellum. Too much movement or noise like we find at the gym could also overstimulate the sensory systems and cause brain fatigue. If you have trouble from one of these factors, it's a good clue that the related brain area needs help.

At some point, the type of exercise that tires the brain may be helpful in rehabilitating that area. Just like with muscles, though, you don't want to overwork an injured area. You need to let some healing take place first, then slowly ease into it. Neuro-physical therapists, chiropractic neurologists, functional neurologists, and vestibular therapists are very good at recommending the right exercise at the right time.

Chapter 32

A Note on Functional Medicine

It could be argued that what is now labeled functional medicine is both the oldest and newest approach to health. Simply put, functional medicine looks at your body as a whole. It identifies weaknesses or dysfunction in individual systems of the body or the interaction between them. Finally, it seeks to improve health through diet, lifestyle, supplementation, and sometimes medication by supporting and strengthening the systems involved.

Functional medicine tries to identify systemic weaknesses before they become pathological, resulting in a named disease. Functional medicine practitioners often use blood tests similar to those used by medical doctors, but the normal ranges are not as generous because they are looking for reduced function.

Functional medicine is not part of a particular degree program or license scope of practice. A wide range of practitioners may take a functional medicine approach to health including, medical doctors, chiropractors, acupuncturists, homeopathic doctors, osteopaths, and nutritionists. Of course, each profession is limited by its own scope. A chiropractor cannot advise you on medications, but if their state allows it, they can advise on supplements.

A great deal of the information in this book comes from the functional medicine approach. When we talk about the brain, how it's injured and how that affects its function, we are talking about one system. We can look at brain injury and take steps to affect the brain directly, but there may be other systems involved. These other systems may or may not have been functioning well before injury. If they weren't, they may be part of the reason it has been hard for you to recover. If they were, the injury to your brain may have an impact on those other systems. That reduced function may, in turn, makes it harder for your brain to recover.

The brain is a big part of the nervous system. Injury to the brain will almost always affect other parts of the nervous system. Different systems that can be affected by mTBI or impact mTBI recovery are the:

- Digestive system

- Immune system

- Endocrine system (glands that make hormones)

- Cardiovascular system

- Musculoskeletal system

We can say that the nervous system and of course, the brain, are our primary concern and focus. In this book we start with that. We can't forget about the other systems, though, because in the long run, they may be the ones that are impacting the brain's function.

Chapter 33

Regulate your Blood Sugar

Summary

A steady fuel supply is extremely important for brain function. It's even more important for healing. Most of the time, the brain uses the sugar glucose to produce energy in special parts of each cell called mitochondria. Mitochondria can be damaged by the chemical processes that occur with concussion. Unstable blood sugar can worsen that damage, slow recovery, and contribute to head injury symptoms. Brain trauma can also create sugar regulation problems, which leads to a negative feedback loop.

What to Do

The first step is to recognize if you have a pattern of poor blood sugar regulation (See next section, 33a, for how to determine this). From there you can make dietary and lifestyle changes to improve it.

Why

Poorly regulated blood sugar increases brain inflammation and directly damages brain cells. This comes from the highs and lows in sugar levels as well as highs and lows in chemicals the body releases to try to maintain steady levels. These chemicals are insulin, from the pancreas, and cortisol, epinephrine (adrenaline), and norepinephrine from the adrenal glands.

Personal Reflections

There is a donut shop around the corner from my office. I know the owner well. I could go out of the back of my office, cross an alley and knock on his back door, even after he'd closed, and he'd bring me my "usual," a chocolate cake donut with chocolate frosting. John, the donut guy, likes me so much he always gave me an extra donut. I always thought I'd eat it later, or save it for my wife, but that never happened. For many years I'd get a temporary sugar boost, then crash later, only to want another boost.

After my initial head injuries, I was tired all the time. I would sleep between patients. I took a two-and-a-half-hour lunch because I'd be completely non-functional after eating. My 10 a.m. or 4 p.m. donut, or at least a coffee, would give me just enough of a boost to get me through the rest of the day. I was doing the absolute worst thing I could have done.

After taking my first seminar on head injury and nutrition, I was spending about $100 a week, wholesale, on supplements, and they really helped. But I didn't change my eating habits. I did become conscious enough to realize that I might need to change my diet. I'd had problems with food intolerances in the past, so I thought I better check that out. I went to a nutritionist, and she put me on a gluten- and other antigen-free diet. That helped too, but I still had issues.

After another seminar on brain chemistry, I realized I might have adrenal fatigue, so I took supplements to support my adrenal glands. They made a huge difference. I didn't have to sleep as much after lunch, my moods were better, and my mind was much clearer. Nonetheless, I kept eating donuts. When I thought I was healed, symptoms started coming back. I was still very susceptible to big flare-ups even with a little jarring or bumps to the head.

It wasn't until I noticed that my big toes were starting to go numb after my double donut binges that I started thinking I might have a problem with sugar. Even then, I didn't really relate it to my head injury symptoms. To cut down on sugar, I decided to do the ketogenic diet, in which you eat very few carbs. It was hard at first.

I was very hungry for about a week, and I missed my donuts and sandwiches. Finally, my head truly started to clear, I slept well, and my energy level went up. The benefits far outweighed the donuts. After a while, even the idea of a heavy carb meal just wasn't appealing.

I still want donuts! But I resist (most of the time), and I wonder how much sooner I would have recovered, how much less I would have spent on supplements, how much permanent damage I would not have done to my brain, if I'd learned about the sugar-brain connection earlier. I have done the keto diet three times now. Once for three months, once for a year, then again for three months. My plan is to do it three months a year and eat a fairly low-carb diet the rest of the year. This has served me well.

Science and Specifics

Generally, brain cells convert glucose into fuel (adenosine triphosphate, or ATP), but they can also use ketones, which are made from fat when glucose levels are low. Glucose is sugar that we eat. The body also makes glucose by breaking down other sugars like fructose from fruit or starch from bread, pasta, and starchy vegetables like corn or potatoes. Sugars and starch are grouped together as carbohydrates. The body can also create sugar from protein. Our system is able to store glucose as glycogen and convert it back when needed.

An injured brain needs more fuel but is able to produce less. Just like when one muscle is injured, other muscles around it are recruited to help. When brain cells are injured, the brain cells around it are recruited, but they don't do the job as efficiently. More of them need to work, so more fuel is used up. At the same time, neurons are using fuel to restore their internal balance.

Right after an injury, the brain will use more glucose to try to provide extra energy. This increase in glucose use happens within about eight days of injury and lasts one to two weeks. After that there's a period of time when the brain's ability to use glucose diminishes. This can last a long time depending on the severity of the injury and the age of the injured person. The worse the injury and the older you are, the longer it lasts. [62]

In severe head injury, hyperglycemia, high blood sugar, is a common complication. Hyperglycemia is a predictor of symptom severity and mortality. In these cases, high blood sugar may be caused by surgery/anesthesia, the stress response, inflammatory response, diabetes mellitus, pituitary and/or hypothalamic dysfunction. [63]

In mTBI, there is no risk from surgery or anesthesia unless you have other injuries. The other causes of hyperglycemia (see above) may still play a role, however. A person could have perfect blood sugar regulation before a concussion and develop problems because of the concussion. This is called post-traumatic dysglycemia. People who had diagnosed blood sugar issues or borderline undiagnosed issues before mTBI may be more likely to have longer recovery times or more complications from blood sugar issues, especially if they are worsened by the injury.

Cortisol, produced by the adrenal gland, is a hormone involved in blood sugar regulation, especially at night. It is commonly associated with stress. If you are very stressed, which is likely, since having a head injury is very stressful, your adrenal glands may be overworked. This is called adrenal fatigue. If your adrenals are not able to make enough cortisol at night to convert stored glucose (glycogen) back into glucose, adrenaline steps in to do the job. This is one reason why many people with blood sugar issues will wake up during the night — they have too much adrenaline running through their system. Of course, the injured brain needs sleep to heal. One more reason to balance your blood sugar.

Typically, blood sugar regulation depends on when and what you eat and your activity level. Insulin is the main hormone involved in these patterns. We will look at different patterns in the next section.

33a

Determine your Blood Sugar Pattern

Summary

Learn if you have an issue with blood sugar and, if you do, identify what kind of pattern you have. This chapter will be helpful to all concussion sufferers, especially those with energy or sleep issues.

What to Do

Take a look at the various symptoms associated with the blood sugar patterns below. The most significant symptom is how you react to food; does it make you tired, does it give you more energy, does it make your irritable? When you react, take note of when you're eating and what you're eating. If you have a lot of the symptoms associated with one or more of the patterns, you can suspect that you have a blood sugar regulation issue. To confirm or rule out blood sugar issues you will need to have your blood tested. These tests may include fasting blood sugar, a glucose tolerance test; HbA1c (an indicator of your average blood glucose levels over the last 2-3 months); triglycerides (a type of fat); cholesterol; insulin; and daily cortisol rhythm. Depending on the laws of where you live, these tests can be ordered by various types of practitioners, though I would recommend having the tests read by a functional medicine practitioner.

There are six general patterns of blood sugar metabolism:
1. Normal
2. Hypoglycemic - too little blood sugar
3. Hyperglycemic or insulin resistant - too much blood sugar
4. Mixed pattern - sometimes hypoglycemic, other times, hyperglycemic
5. Type 1 diabetes
6. Type 2 diabetes

Here are the symptoms to look for:
1. Normal

- No symptoms

2. Hypoglycemia

- You depend on caffeine to get started and keep going
- You crave sugar before meals and before bed
- Poor appetite in the morning
- You crash between meals
- You wake up in the middle of the night
- Pale skin
- Blurred vision
- Fast heart rate
- Facial tingling or numbness
- Between meals or if you miss a meal you:
  - Feel shaky, jittery, have tremors
  - Get agitated, nervous, upset easily
  - Your memory gets worse
  - You get lightheaded
  - Your concentration is poor

3. Hyperglycemic or insulin resistant

- Fatigue after meals
- Crave sweets during the day, especially after meals
- Crave sweets even after eating sweets
- Need caffeine after meals
- Have a strong appetite and thirst

- Over-eat large, high-carbohydrate meals
- Have difficulty losing weight
- Have waists bigger around than their hips
- Urinate frequently
- Frequent yeast or skin infections
- Have problems falling asleep
- Wake up tired even if they sleep
- Gain weight under stress
- Slow healing cuts

4. Mixed pattern

- Some hypoglycemic symptoms and some hyperglycemic symptoms

5. Type 1 diabetes

- Extreme thirst
- Frequent urination
- Drowsiness
- Increased apatite
- Sudden weight loss
- Fruity smelling breath
- Brain fog
- Heavy breathing
- Vision changes

6. Type 2 diabetes

- Extreme thirst
- Frequent urination

- Drowsiness
- Increased appetite
- Sudden weight loss
- Blurred vision from dry eyes
- Tingling hands or feet
- Slow healing cuts or bruises, infections
- Urinary tract infections
- Thrush
- Dry itchy skin
- Irritability, mood swings

Why

The brain generates energy using oxygen and either glucose (sugar) or ketones (discussed later). To heal, the brain needs a lot of energy. It's important that the fuel to make that energy is delivered in a smooth, consistent way.

If your blood tests come back and your sugar metabolism is normal, congratulations! You may not need to change your diet or lifestyle. However, having a mild traumatic brain injury can change the way you process sugar, so the dietary and lifestyle advice in the next chapter is still important to you.

If your tests show blood sugar regulation is abnormal, it's important to work with your health care practitioners to understand which pattern you have, how it affects you, and what you can do about it. The endocrine system regulates blood sugar; it includes all the glands and hormones. The parts of the endocrine system that regulate blood sugar are the pituitary gland and hypothalamus in the brain, the adrenal glands, and the pancreas. There is a huge difference between pathological blood sugar issues and functional blood sugar issues. A pathological issue is a disease. If you are having blood sugar regulation issues, consult with your doctor to first rule out the possibility of pathology: type 1 diabetes, type 2 diabetes, cancer, and autoimmune issues. These must be medically managed.

Please note, when having blood tests done, if you are being tested for functional issues, normal ranges are narrower than when testing for pathology. In this way, using functional ranges can detect deficiencies in organ system functions that are affecting your overall health, but have not yet reached a disease state. A result in the low or high normal range on a scale used to diagnose disease, may be outside of the normal range on a scale used to test function. A medical doctor will usually look at tests to rule out pathology. A functional medicine practitioner will look for more subtle deviations from the optimal. Functional issues may respond to diet, lifestyle, or environmental changes, while pathology may also require medication or even surgery.

Personal Reflections

When I first started to learn about how the body uses sugar and what might go wrong, I found it very confusing. You might, too. The truth is that except for the "normal" pattern, every one of these patterns overlaps with at least one other to some degree.

Hypoglycemia can lead to insulin resistance. The mixed pattern is both hypoglycemia and insulin resistance. Insulin resistance can lead to type 2 diabetes. Type 1 diabetics may also have insulin resistance. It's kind of a mish-mosh. As you read about the different patterns one may really "fit" you, but it probably will not be that clear. The important thing is to recognize if sugar is impacting your well-being. From there I would enlist the help of a functional medicine practitioner to use lab testing to help clarify and address that dynamic.

Really, the most important thing is understanding how you relate to sugar in your daily life. I find sugar highly addictive. It makes me feel good, but like every drug, the effect is temporary and in the long run, it's damaging. We need sugar to live; the brain needs sugar to produce energy and even more sugar to heal. The issue is how do we provide the brain and body with that sugar? It needs to be done in a way that meets the needs of the body but doesn't produce spikes in the level of sugar or insulin in the blood.

Science and Specifics

The most common indicator for blood sugar metabolism problems is a change in your energy level after eating — either an increase or decrease. Another very common symptom is sleep issues.

Functional Reactive Hypoglycemia

Functional reactive hypoglycemia, which is different from hypoglycemia, is a condition in which one common symptom is getting a boost of energy after eating. This means you have drops in your blood sugar levels that rob you of energy, so when you eat, you get a little boost. This is why you may like high-sugar snacks, including fruit, throughout the day.

Some hypoglycemia symptoms are also concussion symptoms, but low blood sugar will make them worse.

People that are hypoglycemic tend to have poor sleep patterns. They haven't stored enough glucose as glycogen to be converted back for nighttime use. The hormone that makes this conversion happen is glucagon. Cortisol triggers the release of glucagon. Cortisol is also released when you are under stress. Even if you have the glycogen stores, you may not have the cortisol due to excess stress. This is called adrenal fatigue. Either way, if the body fails to restore glucose levels by breaking down glycogen with cortisol, it has to create glucose from protein, a process which is also done using cortisol and glycogen. If you are out of cortisol, your body will use adrenaline. This can wake you up.

Hypoglycemic people typically don't want to eat in the morning. They just don't feel hungry, or the thought of food may even make them nauseous. This is also due to adrenaline. It puts your nervous system in the "fight or flight," sympathetic state, ignoring the fact that you should be hungry.

Reactive hypoglycemia can lead to a mixed pattern (having both hypoglycemia and insulin resistance) or insulin resistance, which can then lead to type 2 diabetes, but you can also develop any of these without ever having had reactive hypoglycemia.

Insulin Resistance

In contrast to hypoglycemia, if you have a drop in energy after a meal you may have developed insulin resistance. This happens when the cells of the body have too much sugar over and over and they don't want any more. They become resistant to insulin, which normally tells them to take sugar out of the blood to use. The body responds by producing more insulin. The result is too much blood sugar and too much insulin circulating in the blood. To confirm insulin resistance, your practitioner will test fasting blood sugar and HbA1c levels. They also may check for high levels of triglycerides, (a kind of fat molecule), high LDL cholesterol and low HDL cholesterol which are associated with this pattern. Insulin resistance may also happen as a result of concussion. [64] Insulin resistance is also called metabolic syndrome and can lead to type 2 diabetes.

Insulin itself can activate microglial cells in the brain, resulting in inflammation. Also, too much or too little insulin in the blood stream can impact the production of serotonin and dopamine in the brain, neurotransmitters that have a lot to do with mood. This is another reason people with poor sugar regulation have changes in energy levels after eating. Serotonin and dopamine spikes or deficiencies can lead to depression, hopelessness, poor motivation, and episodes of rage. [65]

Lack of exercise will also set you up for insulin resistance. You are not using all those carbs and sugars you've eaten. As insulin resistance gets worse, you may find you're more hungry, thirsty, and tired most of the time.

Mixed Pattern

A mixed pattern is exactly what it sounds like, some hypoglycemic aspects and some insulin resistance aspects. If you tend to have hypoglycemic symptoms between meals and insulin resistance symptoms after meals, you may have a mixed pattern.

Type 1 Diabetes

Type 1 diabetes is a medical condition, a pathology that needs to be medically managed. If you have type 1 diabetes, you probably already know it. Most cases are diagnosed by age fourteen, though some as late as the forties. This kind of diabetes is thought to have genetic and/or autoimmune causes. Either way, the result is that the pancreas cannot produce insulin well enough to regulate blood sugar. This means that you have to monitor your blood sugar and inject yourself with insulin.

Studies have shown that people with type 1 diabetes who have moderate to severe traumatic brain injury have more risk of developing dementia[66] or dying.[67] It's not clear if this is because the head injury makes managing the diabetes more difficult or if the diabetes makes a person's reaction to head injury more severe. Either way, it's important to see that having type 1 diabetes adds a risk factor to moderate to severe TBI and may therefore add risk to mild TBI. If you have type 1 diabetes and have had a concussion, you may need to monitor your blood sugar more frequently and adjust your insulin use under the supervision of a medical doctor.

Type 2 Diabetes

Also called adult-onset diabetes because it's usually diagnosed after someone is forty, type 2 diabetes has both genetic and lifestyle components. That means you're more likely to develop it if you have people in your family who have it, but maybe not if you have a good diet, exercise, and take care to not become overweight. Type 2 diabetics tend to have some insulin resistance as well as decreased insulin production. The result is not being able to get glucose into cells for energy production and having too much glucose in your blood stream. Studies have also shown that people with type 2 diabetes who have moderate to severe traumatic brain injury have more risk of dying, but not as much as those with type 1. [68]

When the blood contains too much glucose, it starts sticking to proteins and fats. This process is called glycation and the molecules the sugar is stuck to are called advanced glycosylated end products, (AGE). These AGE are responsible for a lot of the problems that come with diabetes, such as neuropathies (painful nerves), circulation problems, and blindness. AGE help produce a chemical called iNOS, a form of nitric oxide which is harmful to cells, including brain cells.[69]

Most importantly for those with mTBI, AGE activate microglial cells.[70] This means a person with diabetes may have brain inflammation even before getting a concussion, with activated microglial cells standing by, ready to produce more inflammation when an injury occurs. Type 2 diabetics also tend to be low in magnesium.[71] Magnesium both protects neurons before injury and helps reduce damage after. All these factors and the resulting inability of type 2 diabetics to use glucose efficiently in energy production makes their brains more vulnerable to head injury.

33b

Diet and Blood Sugar

Summary

If you have consulted with your doctor, taken notes on your energy levels before and after eating, and figured out you have an unhealthy blood sugar pattern, you can make changes in your diet to shift to a healthier pattern.

What to Do

Eat to provide a steady flow of fuel to the brain and body. This means avoiding big dips or surges in blood sugar. This is going to look very similar no matter what your current blood sugar pattern is, though there are different challenges along the way for different patterns.

Eat like a type 2 diabetic. That means eating regularly throughout the day. No skipping breakfast. Most people need to eat less sugar and other carbohydrates, and more of a good combination of protein, fiber, and good fats.

Here are the basic guidelines: Eat 3 meals a day. Each meal should include a lean protein, healthy fats, and be low in carbohydrates. Snack between meals on protein-rich foods. Reduce overall carbohydrate consumption. When eating a meal, eat your vegetables and protein first, then the carbs. The result will be lower blood sugar and insulin levels.[72] The easiest way to reduce carbs is to cut out grains, processed foods, dried fruit, fruit juices, and high-carb fruit like bananas and pears, plus alcohol, beans, milk, and, of course, sugar. An added benefit to cutting out grains and dairy is that you may have sensitivities to these foods that trigger inflammation.

If you feel energized after a meal or you get tired and cranky between meals, you have eaten too little throughout the day. If you feel tired after eating, you've just had too many carbohydrates. Of course, it will take time for your body to change, so be kind to yourself and have patience.

If you have made all the dietary and lifestyle changes suggested by your doctor and in this book and you are still having energy changes after eating, you may have food sensitivities or an adrenal gland issue. Low cortisol will look like hypoglycemia, high cortisol will look like insulin resistance. In all cases, you will benefit from the guidance of a health care professional who understands sugar regulation, especially as it relates to head injury.

Why

We know that the injured brain needs more fuel so it may seem odd to eat less sugar and other carbohydrates. The Standard American Diet (SAD) has carbs at the base of the food pyramid. That may be okay for people who work very physical jobs, but most of us simply do not use that much energy, which means the body doesn't process all that fuel properly. Peaks and valleys in the fuel supply contributes to brain inflammation and disrupts hormone and neurotransmitter balance. This can keep an injured brain in a constant downward spiral.

Personal Reflections

One of the biggest shocks for me in the blood sugar maintenance journey has been changing my idea of a "healthy" diet. There are many foods that are healthy, but if you eat too much at once or eat them by themselves or at the wrong time, they can spike your blood sugar or insulin level. I am thinking of things like fruit, fruit juice, root vegetables, high quality breads and pasta. All of these foods have their place if eaten in the right quantity and time with protein and fat, but otherwise, they can disrupt your blood sugar.

Science and Specifics

There are a number of popularized low-carb diets. The Atkins diet was probably the first and most widely recognized. You may have also heard of the ketogenic diet, South Beach Diet, the Paleo diet, the Zone Diet, the Dukan Diet, the Whole30 diet or the ZeroCarb diet. All of these have their merits and place. Sometimes it's nice to have the guidance these diets provide. Going on a diet usually means a temporary program. This can be very helpful, but in the end, the idea is to make a lifestyle change. Generally speaking, eating fewer carbs than you currently are eating is an excellent first step. A guideline for an overall low-carb approach is eating 50 to 100 grams of carbs per day, but the ratio of carbs to protein and fat is also important. You will end up eating more fat, which we've been taught not to do both for weight and heart health; however, if you cut down on carbs, you will start burning that fat for energy. The ratios of fats, carbs, and protein are call metrics or macros. Macros for different diets are calculated based on your gender, body fat percentage, activity level and goals. In terms of calories, a general guide might be about 15 to 30 percent carbs, 40 to 70 percent fat and 15 to 30 percent protein.

This would be a good time to consult a nutritionist. Do a food diary so they can see how you've been eating and create a plan based on your needs. There are many apps you can use both to determine your metrics and track how you are doing. Some are geared more for weight loss, while others are more dedicated to insulin resistance. Apps for people with type 2 diabetes may even include estimates on insulin, HbA1c (a measure of blood sugar levels over time) or blood glucose levels, based on the foods you enter.

Challenges by Blood Sugar Pattern

People with reactive hypoglycemia typically don't feel hungry at breakfast so they don't eat it. But, as you've undoubtedly heard before, skipping breakfast isn't good for your body. It deprives your body, in general; it deprives you of brain fuel; and it perpetuates the hypoglycemic pattern. So sorry, you have to eat breakfast. (One exception to this is intermittent fasting, covered later, but not for those in a hypoglycemic pattern.) The good news is that if you can change your eating habits, in time, you will rest easier at night and wake up wanting to have breakfast. The added sleep and steady flow of energy will help your brain heal. If you find yourself crashing between meals, have a protein rich, low-carb snack and move your body a little.

A challenge for the type 1 diabetic is avoiding the trap of relying completely on insulin injections and medication to regulate blood sugar without also managing it through diet. In doing this, you may be able to keep within ranges medically, but spikes in blood sugar and insulin are damaging to the brain and body. It's important to know that a person with type 1 diabetes can also develop insulin resistance. One sign of this would be needing more and more insulin to regulate blood sugar levels.

People who have insulin resistance or type 2 diabetes tend to really enjoy eating and drinking. There is a reason that comfort foods are generally full of carbohydrates; they make us feel full and content, satisfied and relaxed. There is also a very gratifying social element of having a big meal and drinks with friends and family. It's hard to deny oneself this kind of pleasure. However, you need to keep in mind that by eating a lower-carb diet, you will be giving yourself a different pleasure: more energy throughout the day and a healthier, clearer mind that will stay with you longer as you age.

No matter what your blood sugar pattern, it may be hard to resist the high-carb snack or meal. Sugar is like a very powerful drug. It will give you a burst of energy or put you in a nice drowsy relaxed state, but it comes with a price. That price is dependence. Each energy boost comes with its very own low. You turn to more sugar or caffeine to recover. Your fuel supply continues to spike and then crash, along with insulin levels perpetuating brain inflammation and postponing healing. It's a trap, but it's one you can find your way out of.

33c

The Ketogenic Diet

Summary

A ketogenic diet provides many special benefits for the head injured. Keto is a high-fat, low-carbohydrate diet that creates chemicals in your body called ketones, an alternate fuel to glucose and fat. There are also potential side effects of the diet to be aware of and prepared for.

What to Do

To do a keto diet, your intake by calories should be about:

70 percent fat

25 percent protein

5 to 7 percent carbohydrates

The easiest way to track this is with one of the many apps you can download to your phone. You will find yourself eating lots of avocados, eggs, bacon and other meats. There are some great recipes for almond pancakes and waffles. You can even make pizza dough out of cream cheese and mozzarella. I sometimes found myself not eating enough protein in which case chicken and fish or even a simple protein powder like gelatin powder can help you meet your metrics.

If you go on the keto diet, I recommend giving it one month. It's a challenge, but if you're able to do it well, you may benefit so much that you want to continue.

The keto diet has become fairly popular for weight loss, energy, and overall brain health; a fair bit of information about it is available in books and online. Not all of it is reliable, but if you're looking for a keto recipe or diet plan, they are very easy to find. There are also many products that are branded as keto because they are low-carb or high-fat. Please know that nothing is off limits in the keto diet, you can eat anything you like; you just need to stay within your metrics.

The goal with the keto diet is to go into ketosis; this is when your body is converting fat into ketones for energy. To know if you are in ketosis, you can monitor your urine or blood. At first you will spill ketones into your urine, which you can measure on urine strips. After a few days or a week, as your body shifts from using glucose for energy to using ketones, you will have fewer ketones in your urine. This is called becoming keto-adapted. Becoming fully keto-adapted may take one to three months.

To monitor your blood, you can buy a device similar to what diabetics use to monitor their blood glucose. In fact, most of the devices can monitor both glucose and ketones, you just need different strips to put in the monitor. You have to prick your finger to get a drop of blood, put it on the strip, and then the machine tells you your ketone or glucose level.

Some sites say a certain level of ketones in the blood is a "nutritional level" or "therapeutic level" but don't worry about that. As long as you're producing any ketones, you are in ketosis. Your levels may be as low as 0.1 mmol/l. That doesn't mean that is all you are producing, it's just what is available in your blood at that moment. The rest you have produced is being used. If your levels are consistently very low, you may be going in and out of ketosis, which means you may need to adjust your metrics or stop cheating.

When you start on the keto diet, you may experience something called the "keto flu." This comes from losing a lot of electrolytes. It feels like the flu without a fever. The easiest thing you can do to avoid this is to season your food with sea salt or another naturally mined salt, which contains lots of minerals.

Another downside of the keto diet is that it can cause constipation. To help with this, you can increase your fiber intake with psyllium seeds, flax seeds, or chia seeds. Try to have the little carbs you are eating be from fruit and vegetables. A daily Vitamin C supplement also helps and there are laxative teas that are quite effective. As always, drink plenty of water.

Why

Ketones are a more efficient and cleaner-burning raw material for brain cells to make fuel, ATP. Becoming keto-adapted and then continuing to use ketones as a raw material for fuel reduces neuroinflammation and bodily inflammation, thereby reducing post-concussion syndrome symptoms. Lowering your blood sugar can also reset your sensitivity to insulin. In some cases, it can reverse insulin resistance or type 2 diabetes.

Ketones are also what's called a signaling molecule. They increase parasympathetic tone in the nervous system, making you more relaxed. The parasympathetic nervous system is associated with healing, rest, and digestion, as opposed to the sympathetic nervous system, which associated with a fight/flight state of stress. They stimulate mitochondria growth in cells, which produces energy. They also stimulate the release of a hormone that promotes nerve growth. Finally, a ketogenic diet allows for a process called autophagy to occur. Autophagy is the body's way of breaking down tangled proteins and damaged cell parts so their components can be re-used.

Personal Reflections

I have done the ketogenic diet three times. Once for three months, once for a year-plus, and then again for about three months. Each time was a big learning experience for me regarding the diet, myself, and humankind, in general.

The first time I tried it, I used urine strips to test ketone production and they never showed anything. I think my body was so happy to have the extra fuel that I never flushed any out. Even when I invested in a ketone blood monitor, my levels were almost always in the 0.1- 0.5 mmol/l range, but I could tell I was in ketosis.

My mind was very clear, scary clear. I almost couldn't keep up with it. I actually adjusted my metrics from 5 percent carbs to 8 percent because I had so much energy, it felt as if I was hopped up on three pots of coffee a day.

Once I turned down the intensity, the time I was on keto was extremely productive. My mind was sharp. I would wake at 5 a.m. refreshed and in a good state of mind, ready to meditate. I was motivated to work and to exercise. All was very good.

So why did I stop? The first time, I was just tired of doing it. We had a vacation planned in Hawaii and I wanted to live it up. It was a disaster. I never had much keto flu symptoms going on the diet, but I think, at least for me, there was a glucose flu from stopping too quickly. I was irritable, confused, and overly emotional. If it hadn't been Hawaii, it would have been the worst vacation ever.

The second time I did the diet, I really got a good pace going. Of course, at first you miss bread, pasta, rice, and sugary fruit, but after a while, I lost my taste for them. Even now that I've been off the keto diet for some time, I can feel how those foods dull my senses and make me feel slow and heavy. They don't interest me much.

I believe that being on the keto diet for a year really reprogrammed my metabolism. My brain is much less vulnerable to flare-ups. That means that a good many of my primed microglial cells have shifted from that M1 inflammatory state to the M2 anti-inflammatory state. Since high school, I would crash after lunch, a classic sign of insulin resistance. That doesn't happen anymore.

The second time I stopped keto, I did it because my cholesterol was literally off the charts; my lab results came back as too high to measure. The research on high cholesterol and keto isn't clear on whether or not it's a problem. To be on the safe side, I went off the diet with the intention of re-checking my cholesterol in six months and possibly going back on it for three months every winter. (Note, it's wise to have your blood monitored by a physician both before and while on a ketogenic diet.)

Why would I go on the diet in winter? I got thinking about how our ancient ancestors must've eaten before farming and domesticated livestock. In the warmer months, carbohydrates are more readily available in nature as fruits, vegetables, and other edible plants. In the fall and winter, root vegetables might be utilized, but not so much.

I believe that we crave carbohydrates because our ancestors needed them to bulk up for the winter months. During winter, when they'd be eating more fish and game, they used the fat on their bodies as an energy reserve. Protein can be converted to glucose, but not very efficiently. The body can use fat as fuel, but the brain cannot. However, fat can be converted to ketones and then used by the brain. I'm not saying that ancient man was in ketosis all winter long, but with two pathways for the brain to create energy, it makes sense to me that the ketogenic pathway would be used more in winter.

In modern society, when every type of food is available pretty much all the time and high-carb comfort food comes in huge portions, there is no check on our drive to bulk up. We can bulk up all year long and a lot of people do. Say hello to obesity, diabetes and heart disease.

When I went off the keto diet the second time, I wasn't very interested in bread or pasta. A blueberry explodes with sweetness when you are on keto. Much more is too sweet and that stays with you for a while. I did, however, fall into a chocolate ice cream habit. Those pounds I lost while on keto came back and more. I was well prepared for winter.

My most recent experience with the diet wasn't as dramatic as the first two. My mind was clearer, but the feeling of being very awake and focused only came a few times in the three months I chose to do the diet. I did sleep extremely well and lost my ice cream belly.

Since going off keto, I chose to continue with a low-carb diet. This is defined as about 15 to 30 percent carbs, 15 to 30 percent protein and 40 to 70 percent fat. It's much easier, to the point that I don't even track what I'm eating. I do not crave carbohydrate -rich foods. On the contrary, the idea of a rice, bread, or pasta-based meal kind of disgusts me. My mental acuity is still good; however, I notice that if I have even a small amount of something that has straight sugar in it, I tend to become irritable. Most interestingly, every time I've checked my ketones, I am still in ketosis. At least for now, I believe I am still keto-adapted.

Science and Specifics

The keto diet has become fairly popular for a number of reasons. It was originally used to treat epilepsy. Now we know it has many more benefits. It can be life-changing for people with insulin resistance and in some cases, type 2 diabetes. Even with type 1 diabetes, going on keto results in a smaller amount of free glucose circulating in the blood, which is good. Those with type 1 diabetes who do the keto diet may run the risk of going into ketoacidosis, with very high ketone levels, and they're also at risk of having high cholesterol levels. [73] Surprisingly, this type of high cholesterol is more related to the conversion process from fat to ketones than it is to the type of fat you are eating. (See Chapters 34 to 36 for more information on fats.)

Doing keto has benefits for the vascular system and has been used to help combat some forms of cancer. Much of the research I refer to here comes from Alzheimer's, mild cognitive impairment, and other neurodegenerative process research. Many people use the diet just to improve their energy levels and mental clarity.

Some people get increases in their LDL cholesterol. These can be short term or more long lasting. In a study of epilepsy patients who got high levels of LDL, they started going back down after a year on the diet or if they went off the diet.

There is growing evidence that a certain type of person on keto gets high cholesterol. They are called Lean Mass Hyper-responders. They tend to be thinner people. Many are endurance athletes.

While LDL may go up, the good cholesterol, HDL also tends to go up. There are many kinds of LDL. Sometimes it is the VLDL, very low-density lipoproteins that go up. These are sometimes called the fluffy LDL and seem to be less of a concern relative to heart disease.

The entire subject of cholesterol and heart disease continues to be the subject of debate. Some say it is not a concern unless you also have high inflammatory markers such as C-reactive protein.

Here are some key points regarding the value of the ketogenic diet for the head-injured:

- After injury the brain uses more glucose for about eight days.
- After that there is a long period in which the brain doesn't use glucose well. How long this period lasts depends on the person's age (the younger you are, the shorter it lasts) and on the severity of injury (the worse, the longer it lasts). [74]
- Ketones can supply up to 60 percent of the fuel used by the brain.
- Making ATP from glucose requires some ATP to get the process started. Making ATP from ketones does not, so the net energy created using ketones is more.
- Ketones stimulate an increase in the number of mitochondria, the part of a cell that makes ATP.
- Making ATP from ketones creates fewer inflammatory reactive oxygen species (ROS), than making it from glucose, so it "burns cleaner."
- Ketones themself are an antioxidant[75] and are anti-inflammatory
- They reduce microglial priming. They convert microglial that are primed from their inflammatory (M1), to their anti-inflammatory (M2) expression. [76]

- On the ketogenic diet, damaged proteins and cell parts are cleaned up and recycled. This is called autophagy.[77] It promotes new nerve connections, (neuroplasticity). Some of the proteins it clears out are associated with Alzheimer's and Parkinson's disease.

- The ketogenic diet improves the microbiome, (bacteria in the gut). That in turn improves blood flow in the brain and the function of the blood brain barrier. [78]

- In long term recovery, the ketogenic diet increases new nerve connections in the hippocampus, which is related to memory, but lowers it in the striatum associated with decision making, reward related behavior, coordinated movement, and sleep regulation. [79]

- Ketones as an energy source reduce the need for insulin and cortisol, both of which are neuroinflammatory.

33d

Intermittent Fasting

Summary

Intermittent fasting can provide many of the benefits of the ketogenic diet or amplify them for those who are keto-adapted.

What to Do

Intermittent fasting is quite simple. Designate periods of time when you eat and others when you do not. The fasting window can be fourteen to sixteen hours, leaving eight to ten hours when you can eat. Basically, it comes down to having an early dinner and a late breakfast. The frequency with which you eat meals is up to you, as long as you leave time for fasting. Some people do it every day, some once a week. Another method involves complete fasting two days a week. I believe this would be too disruptive to the fuel supply for an injured brain, especially if you are not keto-adapted from having been on the ketogenic diet.

Why

With fasting, you will burn fat and produce ketones for fuel. If you are not keto-adapted, you will not be able to use the ketones as well for fuel. Otherwise, you will have all the benefits of being on the ketogenic diet, but less consistently and to a lesser degree. If you are keto adapted fasting will kind of turbo charge the benefits of the ketogenic diet.

Intermittent fasting is being studied as it relates to degenerative diseases of the brain. This is because, like the ketogenic diet, it stimulates autophagy and reduces neuroinflammation. Autophagy is the recycling of damaged proteins and cell parts; it helps clear out the protein amyloid-beta in the brain. This protein is associated with Alzheimer's and Parkinson's, usually referred to as amyloid plaques. These plaques get started in a neuroinflammatory environment. Intermittent fasting also increases BDNF (brain-derived neurotrophic factor), which stimulates nerves to connect and improves memory. [80]

Personal Reflections

The first two times I was on the keto diet, I was afraid to try intermittent fasting. That's because I've had blood sugar issues in the past and would crash hard if I missed a meal, so I didn't know if fasting would leave me exhausted. After learning more about it, however, and normalizing my blood sugar regulation, I made it part of my routine for my third cycle of keto. It really was no problem at all. In fact, I noticed an extra surge in motivation after breaking the fast. Sometimes the surge of energy can be strong, it's like drinking a pot of coffee (and yet much more healthy, of course). I get a lot done, but it can be frenetic.

Having been off the keto diet and on a low-carb diet for several months, I find that an occasional fast day can really boost my mood and productivity. The energy often comes once the fast is broken. It seems that that first bit of food provides an exponential amount of energy.

I've had patients who maintain their eating/fasting windows all the time. I wonder if this routine gives them the benefit of becoming keto-adapted.

Science and Specifics

To start producing ketones, and get the benefits of a fast, you need to use up your glycogen stores in the liver. (Glycogen can be converted to glucose for energy.) That means burning 700-

900 calories of glucose stored as glycogen which takes around 10-14 hours, less if you exercise. For intermittent fasting to be truly beneficial, especially for the head-injured, you should be keto-adapted before you do it. When you're keto-adapted, your glycogen levels will already be low, so they will deplete sooner. You will already be producing ketones and your body will be able to use them well.

If you are not already keto-adapted and have sugar regulation issues when you start intermittent fasting, you will crash. Your blood sugar level will drop. You will produce ketones, but your body will not be set up to use them. You will have no fuel. After you crash, you may have a big blood sugar/insulin spike, doing more harm than good.

Chapter 34

Essential Fats

Summary

The injured brain needs lots of fat. Three kinds of fat are especially important: DHA, EPA and DPA, otherwise known as omega-3 fatty acids or essential fatty acids. They are considered "essential," because our body cannot produce them, so we need to eat them. Omega-3s are found in food, especially fish that live in cold water, such as salmon, cod, anchovies, mackerel, smelt, and tuna, and some in grass-fed lamb and beef. The body can produce EPA and DHA in very limited quantities from another omega-3, ALA, which is plant-based and found in chia and flax seeds, walnuts, and some beans. Considering the quantities the brain needs for healing, the amount of omega-3's we produce or ingest needs to be supplemented in the form of fish oils.[*]

What to Do

Take from 500 mg to 10,000 mg per day of omega-3 fatty acids, primarily DHA.

Why

The brain is about 60% fats. DHA makes up about 40% of that; it's one of the main ingredients of neuron cell walls. DHA also makes up 97% of the omega-3 fatty acids in the brain. DHA is neuroprotective and reduces inflammation. Once the supply is low, the brain will start sacrificing the cell walls of neurons to provide more DHA. This damages or kills those cells, releasing their content into the fluid between the cells, causing more inflammation. The amount of DHA in the brain and the chemicals that help incorporate DHA into the cell membranes goes down after TBI. [81]

Increasing DHA levels in the brain has many benefits. Supplementing before a TBI[82] [83] or right after lessens the damage to neurons and neuron death. It also lowers excitotoxicity[84] and

---

[*] Statements regarding supplements have not been evaluated by the FDA. Supplements are not intended to diagnose, treat, cure or prevent disease.

lessens microglial activation. [85] It helps shift primed microglia from the inflammatory to the anti-inflammatory state. [86] More DHA helps restore levels of chemicals that help neurons connect, so head-injured rats given DHA recovered their ability to learn and remember better than those who weren't given DHA. [87] Even thirty days after injury, DHA helps restore energy production in neurons, reducing ongoing damage.

EPA is very good for general inflammation and cardiovascular health. Since brain inflammation and systemic inflammation are related, decreasing one helps decrease the other. Of course, good circulation is very important to bring oxygen to the brain.

Resolvins are chemicals derived from fats. RvD1 from DHA improves cognitive and motor function after TBI when combined with aspirin. RvE1, from EPA, reduces microglial activation and improves sleep. [88] RvE1 production has also been shown to increase when EPA and aspirin are taken together. [89] Please consult a medical professional before taking even over-the-counter drugs like aspirin.

DPA is getting more attention in research. It is an intermediary between EPA and DHA, which means the body can convert it into either one. It has some benefits of both EPA and DHA for cardiovascular health; it also reduces inflammation and lessens oxidative damage to the brain. [90] Taking DPA with EPA and DHA actually increases the absorption of EPA and DHA and helps balance the omega-6 to omega-3 ratio.

Personal Reflections

DHA is the first supplement I recommend taking after getting a concussion or being re-injured. Many times, someone has come to see me soon after a car accident with a constant headache or mild concussion symptoms. Usually, they don't realize that they've had a concussion and their brain is inflamed. These symptoms often clear out quickly using DHA, chiropractic adjusting, and cranial work. In my opinion, this early use of DHA is very helpful in halting the inflammatory process, saving these people from more severe ongoing problems.

In more chronic cases where neuroinflammation is more advanced, DHA is still an important part of the protocol, though it probably will not be able to resolve symptoms alone.

Because DHA is neuroprotective, I also recommend it even after brain inflammation and symptoms have decreased. At that point, I might recommend a supplement that contains a blend of EPA and DHA.

Finally, I've found it's a good idea to bring DHA and EPA supplements when I travel. I tend to have little flare-ups whenever I travel by air, and it takes me about a day to recover for every new time zone I enter. Essential fatty acids along with a few other supplements get me back on track. I also seem to bump my head more often when traveling, so it's good to have all those supplements in the emergency kit.

Science and Specifics

For overall health and well-being practitioners recommend anywhere from 500 to 5000mg total omega-3s daily usually in a 1:1 or 2:1 ratio EPA to DHA. Recommendations for brain trauma range from 500mg to 10 grams a day, a very wide range. In brain trauma studies the ration of EPA to DHA may go from 1:4 up to 1:100 or just all DHA. It is hard to be more specific because there really is no established dosage. Most studies on head injury and fatty acids are on rats.

Some doctors like to recommend starting low and working up until you get the desired effect. How well you respond will depend on how severe your issues are and what other fats are in your diet. Personally, I would rather start with a relatively high dose. If that provides the desired effect maybe work down, otherwise work up. DHA is expensive, but the cost of letting your brain continue to lose neurons cannot be measured. The only downside to this strategy is that a sudden increase in fat may cause digestive issues. If it does you will have to lessen the dose, let your digestive tract adapt, then increase from there until you benefit.

When you purchase omega-3 fatty acids in the form of fish oil supplements, make sure that you get them from a reputable company. Studies have shown that some fish oil supplements have other fats in them or are oxidized, i.e. rotten.[91] If that's the case, you'd be missing out on one of the omega-3s' main functions, that of antioxidant.

Note, when you first start taking DHA, you may get some of the anti-inflammatory benefits right away, but it takes time for the DHA to be integrated into the cell walls of neurons, so it may be a month before you start to get more benefit.

If you take a high dose of fish oils and get crampy or have a lot of fishy-tasting burps, it could mean that the oil is spoiled or your digestive system is not able to digest fat well. This could mean you have an issue with your pancreas or gall bladder. Reduce what you are taking and let your body adapt before trying to raise it up again. If that doesn't work, get a new bottle or different brand of oils. If you are still having trouble, consult a functional medicine practitioner.

Chapter 35

Eat Healthy Fats

Summary

Our bodies need fat to function. Many different processes depend on fat, and all outer surfaces of every cell in our bodies are made primarily of fat. The kinds of fat in the cell membrane affect how well the cell functions. This is particularly true with brain cells. Every diet recommends eating "healthy fats," but what does that mean? What is too little? What is too much? What kind of fat should you eat?

What to Do

Avoid corn oil or foods fried in corn oil.

Increase the amount of omega-3 polyunsaturated fats in your diet, typically found in fish, eggs, nuts and avocados, and decrease the amount of omega-6s. Do not eat processed foods.

Cook with liquid oils rather than butter or thick oils such as coconut or palm oil. Do not let your oil smoke when sautéing. Olive oil is okay for sautéing in most cases, but if sauteing or frying at high temperatures, it's best to use avocado oil.

Why

Fat is essential for the body. Per Chapter 34, the most important fats for good health, DHA, EPA, and DPA, are called essential fatty acids. Our bodies cannot produce them well so we must eat them. These fats promote brain healing by reducing inflammation and play a key role in the health of individual brain cells.

Personal Reflections

Let's face it, fat is vilified. Why? Because *being* fat is vilified. Yet, fat is very important for health and it's delicious! Fat actually carries the flavor of food. That's why non-fat foods are often full of sugar or flavoring. It's also why people often fail on diets because they end up substituting carbohydrates for the fat they take out of their diet.

Being fat has many health risks but eating fat itself is not inherently bad for you. The key is to eat the various types of fat in the right quantities and proportions. We tend to eat too much saturated fat, found in foods such meat, cheese and other dairy products. The unsaturated fat we eat tends to be more omega-6 than omega-3, for example, fried foods and salad dressing. If you can change the balance of those fats, you will improve your health. Your brain will recover more quickly. Your overall inflammatory load will be less. Your heart and blood vessels will be healthier.

If you are overweight, you may need to change the balance of fats you're eating and lessen the quantity. Losing weight requires using more calories than you consume.

If you do the ketogenic diet, the rules change. You will be eating much more fat; however, you should still try to balance your fats. Since you will be eating very few carbohydrates, the fat you do eat will be used for fuel. If you need to lose weight, eat fewer calories than you burn and the body will burn fat you are carrying for fuel.

Science and Specifics

All oils and fats in food have a blend of the three levels of saturation. For example, we think of fat from meat as saturated because it is solid at room temperature, however, the fat in beef is about half saturated, a little less than half mono-unsaturated, and 4% poly-unsaturated.[92] On the other hand coconut oil, which has become quite popular, is about 81% saturated fat.[93]

Trans Fatty Acids

Trans- or hydrogenated fatty acids, which used to be found in margarine and many processed foods, are very bad for health, especially the heart. In the brain, they get into nerve cell membranes and disrupt many functions, and also cause inflammation. They negatively affect mental performance and have been implicated in depression and Alzheimer's.[94]

Trans-fatty acids are banned from food production in the U.S. and most European countries. Corn oil naturally has 0.25g/100g of trans fat. Frying food in corn oil, especially stir-frying creates more trans-fat.[95] The longer the oil is used, the more trans-fat.

Polyunsaturated Fats: Omega-6 and Omega-3 balance

Polyunsaturated fats are liquid at room temperature. The term poly-unsaturated refers to the chemical structure of the fat. The main two are Omega-3s and Omega-6, but there are many others. Foods that have a lot of polyunsaturated fat may be particularly high in one type, but usually contain many types. Fish, nuts, and vegetable oils are all high in polyunsaturated fats. The essential fats discussed in chapter 34 are all omega-3 polyunsaturated fats. They are considered essential because the body does not produce them well or in enough quantities, so we must eat them. Two other essential polyunsaturated fats are ALA, an omega-3, and LA, an omega-6 fatty acid. The body cannot produce these at all.

ALA can be converted into DHA or EPA which are both anti-inflammatory and play important roles in brain health. Americans get most of the Omega-6 LA from chicken, baked goods, eggs and salad dressing. Oils rich in LA from highest to lowest concentration are grapeseed, sunflower, corn, cottonseed, and soybean. LA can be converted into Arachidonic Acid, AA. Because AA is part of both anti and pro-inflammatory chemical processes some practitioners recommend you avoid all Omega-6s, but the body needs them. The question is, what's the best ratio of omega-6 to omega-3 for the body and brain?

Daily recommended intake of LA in the US for men and women between the ages of 19 and 50 is 17 and 12 grams/day. Less before and after those ages.[96] Meeting these requirements is really easy because there is plenty of Linoleic Acid our diets.

We eat more omega-6 fats than omega-3's; in fact, the ratio in the American diet is estimated to be up to 25:1. According to one theory centered around heart disease, asthma, cancer and inflammatory bowel disease, it's unhealthy to eat too many omega-6s in relation to omega-3s. It's believed that primitive man ate about a 1:1 ratio of omega-6 to 3. The two types of fat compete for space in cell membranes; certain research has shown that too much omega-6 blocks the good effects of omega-3 and causes inflammation. There is still a lot of debate about this idea. Some scientific literature supports the idea[97] some does not. [98]

For the brain, it has been found that a lower omega-6 to omega-3 ratio is a good predictor of better memory, faster learning[99] and "fluid intelligence" in old age. In animal studies, a lower ratio meant lower rates of Alzheimer's. [100] A more balanced ratio could be achieved by increasing Omega-3s without reducing Omega-6, however considering how out of balance we are, it is also a good idea to reduce 6s. A simple way to do this is to avoid processed food as they use a lot of corn and soybean oil. Soybean oil consumption in the US has skyrocketed over the last 20 years. Even now that hydrolyzed soybean oil is illegal to use, it has been replaced by a thicker oil made with a genetically modified soybean. There are about 7 grams of LA in one Tablespoon of soybean oil.

Mono-unsaturated fats

Mono-unsaturated fats come mostly from plant sources; avocado, olive, canola, and nut oils are all mono-unsaturated. For the head-injured, mono-unsaturated fats are preferable to saturated fat because a diet high in saturated fat causes brain inflammation. [101] Mono-unsaturated fats are also considered more heart-healthy than saturated fats (found in coconut oil and dairy products and meat), as they increase your level of HDL cholesterol and lower LDL cholesterol. This is important, especially if you go on the ketogenic diet and are eating a lot of fat. For the head injured these fats are preferable to saturated fat because a diet high in saturated fat causes brain inflammation.

Cooking with mono-unsaturated oils rather than saturated fats is also healthier because they have higher smoke points, which is the temperature at which an oil will start smoking. It's best not to get to that point, as a smoking oil results in oxidation, which causes inflammation and produces carcinogens. Avocado oil has the highest smoke point, at 520 degrees Fahrenheit, (271 Celsius). Extra virgin olive oil is sometimes preferred for its flavor; its smoke point is between 375 and 400, (190-204 Celsius).

Saturated fats

Saturated fats are solid at room temperature and are derived mostly from meat and dairy. They're also found in cocoa butter, as well as palm and coconut oil. One study showed that rats on a high-saturated fat and sucrose diet that were concussed did not produce as much brain derived neurotrophic factor (BDNF), which promotes new nerve connections, compared to concussed rats on a regular diet. The rats on the high-saturated fat diet weren't able to learn as well as the other concussed rats. [102]

This is not to say you must cut out all meat and dairy; saturated fat is still important for health, plus meat and dairy have many other nutrients. But best to eat them in moderation. Again, this is a concern when doing the ketogenic diet. as it's a high-fat diet. You will need to make an effort to replace saturated with unsaturated fats where you can.

Chapter 36

Supplements for Brain Inflammation

Summary

The injured brain has many needs. Primarily, it needs for inflammation to be greatly decreased so you can literally clear your mind. For that to occur, the brain needs to be protected, calmed down, and to become less reactive. It needs to produce more energy, it needs oxygen, and it needs to heal damaged neurons and make new connections. All of these processes have benefits of their own, but in mTBI and post-concussion syndrome, those benefits are secondary to their part in controlling neuroinflammation. In my opinion, neuro-inflammation is the primary driver of ongoing symptoms.

We cannot rely on supplements alone to fulfill all these needs; however, there are many supplements that can help. Statements regarding supplements have not been evaluated by the Food and Drug Administration. They are not intended to diagnose, treat, cure or prevent disease and should not delay or replace other medical treatment. They do help the body do what it naturally wants to do. Thus the name supplement: something that completes or enhances something else when added to it.

What to Do

I would like to be able to recommend how much of each supplement you should take and for how long. Unfortunately, there are no clear standards. Each person is different. Each injury is different. Many of the studies done on supplements were done on animals. Often the dosage is in milligrams per kilogram based on the animals' weight. This doesn't always convert well to humans, who weigh a good deal more than rats. I've offered a few ranges of dosage in the Science and Specifics section, but it's best to have the guidance of a functional medicine practitioner who knows your individual condition and has experience treating post-concussion syndrome.

The supplements in the chart below serve many needs of the injured brain. Many overlap and boost the effects of others.

Instead of trying one, seeing if it works, and then trying something else, it's better to blend them.

The top five supplements listed on the chart: magnesium, DHA, Vitamin D, glutathione, and polyphenol blend are, in my opinion, the most important. Take those that apply to your degree of inflammation. If you're not having symptoms of neuro-excitotoxicity, you may not need magnesium. If you are overly sensitive to sound, light or busy environments, it's a high priority.

	Nerve protection	Excitotoxicity	Acute Inflammation	Chronic Inflammation	Glial Priming	BBB Repair	Circulation	Mitochondria support	Plasticity
Magnesium		✓	✓			✓			
DHA	✓	✓	✓	✓	✓	✓			✓
Vit D	✓	✓	✓	✓	✓	✓			
Glutathion	✓	✓	✓	✓	✓	✓			
Polyphenol blend	✓	✓	✓	✓	✓	✓	✓		✓
Antioxidants									
B2 Riboflavin		✓	✓	✓					
B3 Nicotinamide		✓	✓	✓				✓	
B6 Pyridoxine	✓	✓							
C Ascorbic acid		✓	✓	✓					
Vit A	✓			✓	✓	✓			
Vit E Tocopherols		✓	✓	✓	✓				✓
Short Chain FA				✓	✓	✓			
Nitric Oxide Support							✓		✓
Vinpocetin							✓		
Ginkgo		✓					✓		
Alpha GPC									
ATP for Adenosine									
Acetyl L-Carnatine		✓		✓	✓		✓	✓	
ALA Alpha lipoic acid		✓						✓	
CoQ10		✓						✓	
CBD		✓	✓	✓		✓			

Buy a supplement case that has three boxes for each day of the week so you can load it up once a week. It saves time and mental energy, and you'll never have to wonder if you took your supplements or not. As discussed, for liquid items or those stored in the refrigerator, put a bean in the boxes for when you need to take them as a reminder.

Why

You don't start rebuilding a house while it's still on fire. You don't try to strengthen a muscle when it's torn. Likewise, you can't heal your brain while it's inflamed.

Supplements are a very passive way to dampen brain inflammation. Once you have what you need to take and a routine established for taking them, it requires very little thought or effort. If you're able to clear your mind just a little through supplement use, it will make everything else easier.

Personal Reflections

I first learned about supplements for head injury at a seminar in 2015, twelve years after my initial injuries. The seminar was basically a jumbled presentation of scientific studies on various supplements and the metabolic pathways they affect. It took me two months to sift through the material and figure out what I needed to take, but I'm glad I did.

I stuck with a routine of heavy supplementation for about three months and things really started to change for me. My brain fog started to lift. My cognitive capacity and endurance improved to the point that I was able to seek out other seminars.

Not surprisingly, most seminars on supplementation are put on by supplement companies. At some point, I realized that the formulas I was taking from the first seminar/company didn't actually have everything I needed in the quantities I needed. Once I switched to some other products, I improved even more quickly.

I've come to prefer single-ingredient or at least single-type-of-ingredient supplements. Many companies have a "brain formula" or a "memory formula." I think the idea with these is to have a few main ingredients supported by other ingredients that either help with absorption or somehow amplify the effect of the main ingredient. My impression with the brain formulas and memory formulas is that all the ingredients are in quantities too small to be therapeutic or there will be something in the formula that's a stimulant or an excitatory neurotransmitter that gives the impression that the brain is working better, but it's not really helping it heal.

I personally have used most of the supplements in this chapter and more. I haven't used CBD or a mitochondrial support formula; I think there are safer, better ways to heal. I include them here because they often show up as supplements for concussion. They may be very helpful for some people and I'm sure there will be more research done on both that may prove me wrong.

Science and Specifics

Magnesium

If you read Chapter 8: Understanding Symptoms, you may remember that injury to the brain causes calcium to rush into the nerve cells. This is part of what happens normally when a healthy nerve fires, but in this case, it happens from a different chemical trigger, and the injured nerve doesn't have the energy to pump out the calcium. It becomes overwhelmed and fires too easily and too much. As discussed in Chapter 8, this is called neuro-excitotoxicity. You become hypersensitive to stimulus and the nerves get tired out. This state perpetuates nerve damage and inflammation and is a big source of symptoms.

Magnesium blocks calcium channels in nerves cell walls. [103] Studies have shown, particularly in the acute, early stages of brain inflammation that magnesium lessens brain damage [104] and loss of motor and cognitive functioning. [105] The importance of taking magnesium soon after injury is well recognized, but in my opinion, it can also be useful later if neuro-excitotoxicity is still a factor. I usually have a patient go through a bottle of magnesium at the beginning of their care no matter where they are in their recovery. There are many forms of magnesium you can buy; magnesium L-threonate is appropriate for brain issues as it can cross the blood brain barrier and easily be transported through the cell walls of neurons.

Magnesium is also helpful in reducing permeability of the blood brain barrier. [106]

Calcium

If you've been advised to take calcium for a specific medical condition, continue doing so, otherwise do not take calcium. Calcium competes with magnesium for absorption in the intestine. [107]

Docosahexaenoic acid (DHA)

DHA is an essential fatty acid. That means that our bodies cannot produce it. Most of our dietary DHA and EPA, another essential omega-3 fatty acid, comes from fish and can be taken in a fish oil supplement. If you are a vegetarian, you will need to supplement with microalgae.

DHA is a major part of the cell membranes of brain cells. DHA provides many benefits to the head injured. Taking DHA before injury, (or re-injury) lessens nerve damage. Supplementation with DHA after TBI increases energy production in the brain and reduce nerve death. It lessens excitotoxicity and dampens several inflammatory chemical pathways. It protects the blood brain barrier, and it even helps with building new nerve connections.

I consider DHA the 1 supplement to take for concussion and post-concussion syndrome. Recommended doses really vary; anywhere from 800mg to 3 grams. Please read Chapter 34: Essential Fats, for more information on DHA and other fats. Also, when supplementing with a lot of essential fatty acids such as DHA, it's important to take other antioxidants to prevent the fats from becoming oxidized before they can do their intended job.

Vitamin D

Deficiency in vitamin D before TBI is associated with worse symptoms. Supplementation with vitamin D after TBI has reduced symptoms.[108] Vitamin D reduces inflammation[109] and excitotoxicity[110] in a number of different ways. It lowers the production of the chemical iNOS, which damages mitochondria (the energy-producing part of the nerve cell). It lessens the glial cells' production of chemicals that trigger more inflammation and increases the glial cells' production of chemicals that decrease glial cell activation. [111] That is, it helps shift primed microglia cells from the M1 to the M2 expression. Vitamin D also helps with magnesium absorption[112] and rebuilding the blood brain barrier.

Vitamin D is my 2 supplement for mTBI after DHA. You can see that it helps at every level of inflammation in multiple ways. It's also rather inexpensive. A small bottle of liquid Vitamin D can last many months. I take it on an ongoing basis for its neuroprotective qualities. The recommended daily allowance for vitamin D is 600iu, 800iu for those over seventy. The National Institute for Health lists the upper limit for vitamin D as 4,000iu/day. A therapeutic dose would be somewhere in the middle.

Glutathione (GSH)

This is the most powerful antioxidant produced by the body and is very important in the protection of the brain and blood brain barrier. Like all antioxidants, it neutralizes the inflammation-producing reactive oxygen species (ROS), also known as free

272

radicals, which are produced in the natural course of all cells making fuel. In the injured brain, inflammation produces much more ROS; it overwhelms the available glutathione's ability to contain it, so it causes more damage and neuroinflammation. The amount of glutathione in the brain goes down as demand for it goes up.

Glutathione can cross the blood brain barrier and is protective for both nerve cells and the barrier. [113] There is also evidence that oral glutathione helps rebuild the intestinal barrier, which can be weakened by head injury and plays a big part in recovery. [114]

Glutathione is available in several different forms. Plain glutathione is not well absorbed.[115] Liposomal glutathione is absorbed into the bloodstream and increases immune response[116], but may not be well absorbed into cells. S-Acetylglutathione, (S-GSH) is well absorbed into the blood and cells. [117] Unfortunately, it can be expensive, but it's worth it. There are supplements that will help put used glutathione back into action. These include selenium, N-acetyl L-cysteine, Cortyceps extract, Gotu-kola extract, milk thistle extract, L-glutamine and ALA.

You can give your body raw materials to make glutathione. These are whey protein and N-acetylcysteine (NAC). Both of these provide cysteine, a building block of glutathione. This may be a less expensive route, but there are drawbacks. The body has to use energy to create the glutathione and whey protein is a dairy product. Dairy can be inflammatory, especially if you have developed intolerance to it. Also, cysteine can be used to make other things and is only used to make glutathione when cysteine levels in the cells are low.[118] Best to go with the actual glutathione supplement.

Polyphenols

Another very important class of compounds for dampening brain inflammation is polyphenols, which include a subgroup called flavonoids. The most effective are curcumin, from the turmeric plant root, and resveratrol, from grapes with Catechins from green tea extract being a close third. There are many others, including: Apigenin, from celery and parsley; pomegranate extract; Rutin from citrus fruits; Baicalein; Baicalin and Wogonin from the herb skullcap; Luteolin; quercetin; Genistein; Hesperetin; and epigallocatechin-3-gallate. These are all available in capsule form often as a blend which is good because to get a therapeutic dose of any one of them would require eating mass quantities of the food they are derived from.

All of the polyphenols are antioxidants and protect the cell mitochondria. Some can reduce neuro-excitotoxicity or brain swelling. [119] Some increase the level of chemicals that augment nerve connectivity and plasticity. Cocoa, blueberry, quercetin and curcumin flavonoids increase blood flow in the brain and may even help grow new blood vessels. [120] What's really special about them is that they can downregulate primed glial cells from the M1 to the M2 expression. [121] This is major if you have ongoing post-concussion syndrome with flare-ups because your microglia are hypervigilant.

For flavonoids to work three things need to happen:

- They have to be activated by the microbiome[122] (the good bacteria that live in your intestines).
- They have to pass through the gut barrier.
- They have to passively diffuse through a healthy BBB.

Different gut bacteria activate different flavonoids,[123] so it's important to have a diverse gut biome. You need to eat a variety of plant fiber from a wide range of vegetables to have a diverse gut biome. Flavonoids themselves actually help promote biome diversity. It may take a while to do that, so it may seem like the flavonoids aren't helping, but give it time.

The gut barrier and the blood brain barrier both need to be healthy for the flavonoids to get to the microglial cells and downregulate them. Flavonoids help repair both the gut[124] and brain[125] barriers. So again, it may take some time, but keep a variety of flavonoids on the job and you should see some results.

Because it may take some time to feel the benefits of flavonoids, you may want to start with a high dose until you notice a change. Then you can taper down as long as you feel the benefit. Other strategies recommended by your functional medicine practitioner to improve gut and BBB health may hasten this process. In my practice, I may start a patient with as high as 1000mg, three times a day.

Other Antioxidants

Antioxidants neutralize ROS (aka free radicals), which damage nerve cells and can cause inflammation. DHA and glutathione are very powerful antioxidants, but there are others that participate in important chemical processes in the brain and body and can therefore be very helpful. These include Vitamins A, C, E, B2, B3, B12 and Selenium. B6 itself is not an antioxidant, but contributes to the effectiveness of Glutathione. [126] B6 also has neuroprotective effects and reduces neuro-excitotoxicity through other mechanisms. [127] Vitamin E dampens neuroexcitotoxicity[128] and reduces microglial activation. [129] Vitamins E and C may shift primed glial back from an amoeboid shape to their original ramified shape and "deactivate" them. [130]

Most of these should be found in a good multi-vitamin. There are some multis available that do not contain calcium. Men's multis generally contain less calcium.

Short Chain FA

Another way to convert M1 to M2 microglia is through short chain fatty acids[131] [132]. We produce our own SCFAs when the microbiome metabolizes fiber. This is another reason to have a diversity of plant fibers in your diet: to support a diverse microbiome. Taking SCFAs as a supplement also helps heal the gut and restore the microbiome.

So, flavonoids and short chain fatty acids like butyric acid, acetate, and propionate are both like fuel that fixes the vehicle that uses the fuel. [133]

Nitric Oxide Support

Nitric oxide species are substances produced by the muscles when we exercise. One of them, nNOS (neuronal nitric oxide species), helps the coordination centers of the brain and the muscles' nerve activation. And eNOS (endothelial nitric oxide species) helps regulate blood flow to the muscles and brain and helps muscle and brain cells create energy.

Technically, supporting nitric oxide production doesn't directly reduce brain inflammation. It is meant more to increase brain circulation, and increasing brain circulation will, in turn, help reduce inflammation.

One more type of NO is iNOS, (inducible) the bad one. It breaks down muscles and joints and has been linked to depression, increased stress response and fatigue.

You cannot supplement with nitric oxide (NO) but you can supplement to increase your levels of NO. You don't, however, want to increase iNOS. All three types need arginine, but when you are inflamed, the arginine tends to be used to make iNOS, especially with high intensity weight training. Do not supplement with arginine.

Nutraceuticals that increase brain circulation through eNOS support are adenosine found in ATP, [134] Vinpocetine, acetyl L-carnitine and alpha GPC, (L-alpha glycerylphosphorylcholine), a precursor of acetylcholine. Gingko biloba supports eNOS. Another supplement that improves brain circulation through other mechanisms is Feverfew.

To really get the benefit of these supplements, it's best to exercise right after taking them. Exercise stimulates nitric oxide production and activation, putting the supplements to work and increasing brain circulation.

Mitochondrial Support

I want to just touch on mitochondrial support here because you will see mTBI protocols that focus very heavily on that. While it's true that a key part of the problem with neuroinflammation is mitochondrial damage, I think we need to look at the cause of the damage first and solve those issues.

If you have neuro-excitotoxicity, one way to dampen it is to can supplement with acetyl L-carnitine, ALA, and CoQ10 to support the mitochondria that are not damaged. This will give the neurons more energy to pump out the excess calcium, which lessens neuro-excitotoxicity and speeds up overall recovery. But I believe blocking calcium from entering the neuron with magnesium is a much more effective, and much more *cost* effective, way to handle neuro-excitotoxicity. Once you are out of the excitotoxic state, controlling and dampening neuroinflammation, in general, will protect the mitochondria. I think it's more effective to use other supplements from above to decrease brain inflammation. Once the fire in your brain is controlled, then start rebuilding.

Cannabidiol (CBD)

Cannabinoids (CBD) are neurotransmitter chemicals that have been has been shown to have a neuroprotective effect in mTBI by reducing neuro-excitotoxicity, neuroinflammation, microglial activation, and blood brain barrier degradation. [135] They are produced by the body but can also be obtained from the marijuana plant.

One issue with CBD products is purity. Researchers use pure CBD. Since it's extracted from the marijuana plant there may be THC in products that you can buy. THC has negative effects on brain function, (see Chapter 17: Don't Smoke Pot). CBD products are classified into:

- Isolate - pure CBD
- Full Spectrum - contains all the cannabinoids in marijuana including THC
- Broad Spectrum - contains multiple cannabinoids excluding THC

The smallest detectable amount of THC is 0.02%, so even the isolate and broad spectrum may have some. Whether it's enough to cause harm to the head-injured is difficult to say.

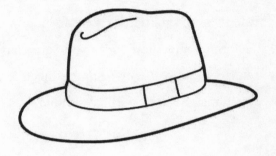

Part 7

Bodily and Brain Inflammation

Summary

Neuro-inflammation can create general bodily inflammation and vice versa, increasing the severity of head injury and prolonging recovery. Inflammation from bodily injuries and digestive system issues participates in an ongoing feedback loop between the brain and body. If you are having continuing symptoms related to both the brain and either the musculoskeletal or digestive systems, this part will have value for you.

Why

Sometimes we focus on one problem at a time in our lives, especially when we have limited energy. If one problem is perpetuated by another, however, nothing gets solved unless both problems are addressed. You may be doing all the right things to lessen brain inflammation, but if you have chronic inflammation from injuries or you have gut issues that are creating inflammation, you may be fighting a losing battle.

Personal Reflections

As a chiropractor who does cranial work, after my initial concussions, my first instinct was to seek the help of a chiropractor and a cranial specialist. They helped quite a bit with my bodily symptoms (such as neck pain and tension headaches) and a little with cognitive symptoms, but the cognitive symptoms kept coming back. The missing part for me was dealing with the brain inflammation. After I learned about and used the nutritional and lifestyle strategies discussed in this book, my cognitive symptoms improved quite a bit, but they were easily brought back by even slight jarring motions to my body. It was only by returning to address issues in my body again through chiropractic and cranial work that I was able to become more stable overall.

Science and Specifics

Musculoskeletal-based inflammation tends to be associated with pain or muscle tension, but not always. Inflammation from the digestive system may be associated with regularity issues or reactions to certain foods, but not always.

In the "not always" situations, these areas may be overlooked. The force required to cause concussion is strong enough to cause injury to other parts of the body; post-concussion, it's worth taking a look at both of these systems even if you don't notice symptoms. In Part 7, we'll look at how neuro-inflammation and general bodily inflammation are connected.

Chapter 37

Healing the Musculoskeletal System

Summary

If your body was injured when your brain was injured or you had pre-existing musculoskeletal issues, they may be contributing to ongoing cognitive or emotional symptoms. In this chapter, we first look at the skull and jaw, and then the spine and the muscles; how they might be involved and how to heal them.

What to Do

Restore proper function of the head and body's joints and muscles by restoring movement and alignment. Reduce physical stress on the nervous system. Reduce bodily inflammation, which perpetuates brain inflammation. Restore the flow of blood and cerebrospinal fluid (CSF) in and around the brain.

Why

It's impossible to separate any one system of the body from another. They are all related and affect each other. The brain, cranial nerves, spinal cord, and spinal nerves are connected to the entire body. Our bones and muscles are moved by the nervous system, but they also house and protect the nervous system. Problems with one system will create problems with the others.

37a

The Skull and Jaw

Summary

The skull and jaw both have a constant subtle rhythmic motion that can be changed by a concussion. Problems in this system can show up as headaches, sinus congestion, balance issues, tinnitus, sleep apnea, snoring, teeth clenching or grinding, jaw popping or locking, and teeth that do not come together well.

What to Do

If you're having problems with your skull and jaw, you'll need to see a health care professional who specializes in cranial therapy and jaw work. The types of professionals who do this work are cranial osteopaths, some Sacro-occipital chiropractors (SOT), and craniosacral therapists. You can find cranial osteopaths and SOT chiropractors on www.concussionprofessionals.com. While there are some extremely gifted craniosacral therapists, the depth of knowledge and experience tends to be greater with doctors of osteopathy and chiropractic.

No matter what the specialty, you should ask the practitioner about his or her degree of knowledge and experience with cranial work, concussion, and TMD (temporomandibular disorder, aka craniofacial pain disorder). The practitioner should take a thorough history of your injury, symptoms, and what you've already done to treat them.

While cranial work can be very relaxing, jaw work inside the mouth can be quite uncomfortable. Also, any cranial work, as all body work, has the potential to bring up emotional responses. It's important that you maintain good communication with your provider both during and after treatment to let them know your personal tolerances. Sometimes less is more. You may benefit from a shorter or less ambitious treatment that you tolerate well, versus an extensive treatment that feels overwhelming and leads you to resist physically or emotionally.

Often after a cranial treatment, a patient will feel very relaxed, tired, or even a little disoriented or dizzy. Take some time after each treatment to get grounded before moving on.

Why

It's important to have healthy skull and jaw movement to insure the flow of cerebrospinal fluid (CSF) around the brain and spinal cord. CSF delivers nutrients to the brain and clears out toxins. CSF also contains some neurotransmitters, creating part of the environment in which the central nervous system functions.

Personal Reflections

It seems odd that in most evaluations of concussion and post-concussion syndrome, the only examination of the head itself is done by machines that take static images. It's well documented that our skull bones move and that CSF flows around the brain and spinal cord. This can only be evaluated by actually touching the head. You would think that practitioners who don't do cranial therapies or treat the jaw would refer to those who do more often. This speaks to one of the downsides of specialization.

I don't believe any one person can grasp the full complexity of the human body; that's why we need to divide it up and specialize. No matter their expertise, doctors of all kinds are taught to look at a patient's history, symptoms, and exam results and come up with a list of possible diagnoses. Even so, the tendency is to look at an issue though one's own lens. As the saying goes, to a carpenter, everything needs a nail.

This can be true for any type of doctor. Your neurologist might not recommend cranial therapy, and your cranial therapist might not recommend a neurological consult. Even clinics that treat only concussion may have their own specific methods they focus on without considering other approaches that may also benefit you. As hard as it is with a concussion, as a patient, it's important to educate yourself and ask questions. Beware of the practitioner who claims to have the solution to all of your needs. Also, beware of those who say there is no solution, that simply means that they have nothing to offer.

Science and Specifics

The brain and spinal cord are surrounded by a type of tissue called dura. The dura attaches to the internal surface of the skull and the sacrum at the bottom of the spine. Think of the dura like a bag that contains the central nervous system and the CSF. Special structures in the dura around the brain filter blood to create the CSF, and other structures allow CSF to go back into the blood stream. It's theorized that this exchange of fluid creates variations in pressure, which causes our skull bones and the sacrum to move in a very specific pattern, sloshing the CSF around the nervous system. [136]

Our jaw bones participate in this subtle movement, but of course they have their own movements of opening and closing. The temporomandibular joints (TMJs) are rather complex joints; they include a disc of cartilage between the mandible, the bone that houses the lower teeth, and the temporal bone, the bone under the ear. This disc and the muscles and ligaments that control the jaw all have to move in synchrony for the mouth to open evenly. If they do not, the jaw may move from side to side, you may get popping or locking, or your teeth may not come together properly.

These issues can cause other problems, the least of which is pain in the jaw. Because the TMJs are so close to the ears, inflammation can spill over and contribute to tinnitus (ringing in the ears) or vertigo (dizziness). A lot of proprioceptive information also comes from the jaw. If the teeth are not coming together properly, it can affect balance.

Muscle tension in the chewing muscles from trying to correct these issues can cause tension headaches or limit the cranial motion and the flow of CSF. Muscle tension can also come from clenching or grinding the teeth while sleeping or during the day, a practice which typically occurs due to stress. I also believe that clenching and grinding can be an unconscious attempt to jump start the cranial motion by squeezing the head with the chewing muscles.

Another consideration with the jaw position and the shape of the pallet is the airway. If your jaw is retruded or your pallet is narrow, it may interrupt your breathing, especially when lying down. One indicator of this is snoring; the worst case is sleep apnea. The result is that you don't get as much oxygen as you need. The brain is the main consumer of oxygen, especially the healing brain. In cases where the bite is significantly off or the airway is limited, cranial therapy may not be enough; you may also need a functional dentist to help expand the palette or change your bite. This should be done in conjunction with aligning the pelvis, spine, and skull by a qualified cranial osteopath or Sacro-occipital chiropractor, many of whom have relationships with functional dentists that do this work.

37b

The Spine and Pelvis

Summary

The spine and the pelvis are closely related to the skull and brain; spine and pelvic issues, especially in the neck, can affect nerves and mimic or increase concussion symptoms such as cognitive or visual dysfunction, headaches, head pain, or dizziness.

What to Do

For the spine and pelvis area, you'll need to consult a professional, though there are more options (than with the skull and jaw) on what type of provider to consult, and more opportunities for self-care. It's safe to say that most people who've suffered trauma to their brain have also had trauma to their spine, especially the cervical spine (the neck). It's also possible that misalignments or motion deficits in the spine that might not have been symptomatic before a concussion could become worse or slow down concussion recovery.

Post-concussion, have your spine evaluated by an osteopath or chiropractor even if you're not having neck or back symptoms. Minimal treatment may make a big difference. If you're having bodily pain, limited range of motion, headaches, head pain, dizziness, or cognitive or visual issues, you may need a series of treatments. A qualified practitioner will evaluate not just your spine but your whole biomechanical frame. If you are receiving cranial therapy, the same person should be looking at the rest of your structure.

In the Skull and Jaw chapter we learned a little about cranial osteopaths and Sacro-occipital chiropractors. Other structural experts that are particularly helpful in the case of concussion are upper cervical chiropractors and chiropractic neurologists. More about these in the Science and Specifics section below.

Why

The acceleration of the brain needed to cause a concussion is between 60-160 g. One g is the force of gravity. Whiplash injuries can occur at accelerations of 4.5 g. Therefore, if you have a concussion, it's highly likely that you have a cervical spine injury as well.

Neck injuries can result in many of the same signs and symptoms as concussion, including headaches, dizziness, and even cognitive and visual dysfunction. This makes it hard to know if these symptoms are coming from the head or neck or both. [137]

Because the entire frame is interrelated, alignment or motion issues in the spine and pelvis can cause issues in the skull and jaw and vice versa. Inflammation due to spinal injuries can also contribute to brain inflammation and vice versa.

Personal Reflections

You'd think, as a chiropractor myself, I would have known about spine and pelvic care as related to concussion, before my injuries. However, if courses on topics such as Sacro-occipital technique, upper cervical techniques, and chiropractic neurology are taught at a chiropractic college, they're usually offered as electives or explored in extracurricular clubs. To truly become proficient in any of them, a doctor must take many post-graduate seminars and spend many hours studying and refining their chosen technique.

This kind of knowledge gap can create the same kind of blind spots that exist in other areas of specialization. As an SOT (Sacro-occipital technique) chiropractor, my first instinct was to be treated by SOT chiropractors and osteopaths. This was very helpful for me, but it didn't take me all of the way. Once I began seeing an upper cervical chiropractor, I made much more progress.

Sometimes when I'm talking with someone who isn't a patient, they may say, "I went to a chiropractor and it didn't help." The belief is that all chiropractors do the same thing. This is understandable because they have only experienced one type of chiropractic, but there are many more. For concussion, I would urge you to see an osteopath, SOT chiropractor, upper cervical chiropractor or chiropractic neurologist. You may even be like me and see one of each.

Science and Specifics

Many different methods are used to treat the spine. All chiropractic methods focus on removing interference on the nervous system by restoring proper spinal movement and alignment. How that is done varies greatly. One method may fit you and your needs better than another. Osteopathy is also focused on restoring movement of the bones, but for the purpose of restoring the flow of fluids, (blood, lymph, CSF), which in turn restores nerve connectivity to tissue. [138]

The primary treatment method of chiropractors is the chiropractic adjustment. This is defined as a high-velocity, low amplitude thrust to restore joint movement or position and remove stress from the nervous system. It's a very specific, quick little push that in some methods requires very little force. The key for the concussion patient is, "very little force." Your brain and spine are already traumatized and on high alert, ready to become more inflamed with additional trauma. Your tolerance level is low, and you should not be receiving adjustments that are delivered with a lot of force. Your chiropractor or osteopath should know this, but just in case, tell them that you do not want manual adjustment on your neck until you know you can tolerate them. There are alternatives.

Sacro-occipital chiropractors use a method called cervical stair stepping to restore motion and stability to the neck. This would be considered a mobilization rather than an adjustment. The doctor holds the head and presses down toward your feet. Because of the angle of the joints in the neck, the head should lift up in four distinct steps. If it doesn't, the doctor will move that level in various directions to free up the motion. SOT doctors also have a very non-invasive, gentle method of aligning the pelvis and lower back using orthopedic blocks. The blocks are padded wedges which are strategically placed under the pelvis with the patient laying face up or face down depending on their needs.

Upper cervical chiropractors focus on the relationship between the base of the skull and the first one or two vertebrae of the spine. In each of several different upper cervical techniques, the practitioner evaluates the alignment of the upper cervical area using specialized x-ray views and other methods to determine the precise angle needed to adjust the atlas, the top cervical vertebrae. The different upper cervical chiropractic techniques include NUCCA, Blair, Atlas Orthogonal, Orthospinology, Grostic, Toggle Recoil and Knee chest. You may want to look at videos online of the techniques or ask if you can observe a treatment to decide which technique you would tolerate well.

Chiropractic neurologists use functional neurology to guide their treatment, which may include chiropractic adjustments; neuromuscular re-education exercises; stimulation of the vestibular (balance); auditory or visual systems; and cognitive exercises. The major concept is that input from all the sensory nerves of the body, especially those receptors in the joints of the spine that sense the movement and position of the body, impact the health of the brain. Therefore, brain health can be improved by improving the health of the joints and muscles that are responsible for the movement and position of the body or by stimulating the sensory systems to target specific areas of the brain.

You can find practitioners who specialize in concussion on https://www.concussionprofessionals.com

Chapter 38

Digestive Health

Summary

The health of the brain and health of the digestive system affect each other. Food sensitivities and imbalances in the intestinal bacteria (dysbiosis) are fairly common, which can have an impact on the brain. While not always the case, concussion can create or worsen these issues, which in turn can worsen brain inflammation or create autoimmunity. Many digestive symptoms overlap with post-concussion syndrome symptoms. If you have these symptoms after working hard to reduce brain inflammation and balance blood sugar, the digestive system may be an important piece of the puzzle for you.

Digestive symptoms may include:

- Brain fog
- fatigue
- dizziness
- headaches
- general muscle and joint pains
- irregularity
- skin issues such as eczema
- excessive gas
- bloating

What to Do

Because of the complex relationship between the digestive system, nervous system, and immune system, it's best to consult a professional with experience in treating this dynamic. That would be someone trained in functional medicine or nutrition. Based on your symptoms and eating habits, they may recommend tests to see if you have intolerance or autoimmunity related to specific foods. Then your diet would be changed accordingly, and your digestive system supported through nutritional supplements. The process is generally divided into three steps: rest, repair and restore.

Rest means eliminating foods that cause you problems. Repair means allowing the lining of the gut to heal. Restore refers to building back the microbiome, sometimes called the gut flora, the good bacteria in your intestines that help digest foods. These three steps overlap. Once your gut heals and the microbiome is restored, you may be able to reintroduce some foods to which you were originally sensitive. It's possible you'll need to continue refraining from some food, especially ones that contain gluten, a protein found in wheat and most other grains and is often used in processed foods.

As an alternative to testing, an elimination diet may be recommended with or without nutritional support. During an elimination diet you stop eating foods that people are often intolerant of or that may cause inflammation typically for at least a month,. You then re-introduce foods one at a time to see how you tolerate them.

The most common problem foods are those that contain gluten. The nice thing about cutting out gluten is that it also eliminates a lot of high-carbohydrate foods, which will help with balancing sugar metabolism, and is essential if you are trying the ketogenic diet. Other common foods that cause inflammation are sugar, alcohol, dairy, corn, legumes, eggs, beans, soy, and nightshades (tomatoes, potatoes, peppers, eggplant).

Many people choose to do an elimination diet on their own; doing so allows you to avoid the expense of testing and professional guidance, but you risk missing something. Also, with testing, you have clear objective measurements of what food you react to and how strongly. More importantly, with testing you can save a lot of time. The longer that a dysfunctional relationship between the gut, brain, and immune system goes on, the more it tends to worsen and affect other systems. The sooner you can clear it up, the better.

Why

The brain, gut, and immune system have an intricate relationship. Disruption in any one of them can cause disruption in the other two. Left unchecked, an ongoing pattern of inflammation and an array of symptoms can be created. Worst case, the immune system can destroy healthy parts of your brain and body.

Personal Reflections

Sometimes you see trends in the health field which are a lot like fads. Suddenly lots of people are being diagnosed and treated for the same thing. These diagnoses are usually based on recently discovered biological facts which explain something that could not be explained before. Not long ago, gluten intolerance was a fad.

Since 1953 it's been known that gluten is the cause of celiac disease. In the 1970s and 80s the idea of non-celiac gluten intolerance came into being when people who did not have celiac disease were found to be reactive to wheat, barley, or rye. Celiac disease is a true autoimmune disease in which the immune system attacks the intestines. Celiac disease also has a genetic component. Non-celiac gluten intolerance happens when the immune system reacts to gluten, creates inflammation in the gut, which then causes symptoms and damage.

In 2003 a paper was published by Alessio Fasano indicating that about 1% of the American population has celiac disease. This was much more than previously thought, and it prompted a great deal of attention and research into gluten, celiac disease, and non-celiac gluten intolerance. In the early 2000's health care professionals were inundated with ads for seminars, supplements, and diet plans related to gluten and how it was the root of all ill health. In 2013 the FDA created rules related to labeling gluten-free food and drink, an industry that had grown to $10.5 billion per year.

My point is, there was a lot of hype around gluten. Some of it was warranted, but some was not. A lot of people really improved their health. Others were misdiagnosed and wasted money and effort on gluten-free foods and supplements they did not need. Parts of the medical establishment looked at the gluten intolerance boom and its treatment as quackery. Some still do.

What came out of the gluten "fad" was a lot of research. Most of what was being said about the evils of gluten was proven true. Our understanding of gluten intolerance, other food intolerances, leaky gut syndrome, autoimmunity, and the gut-brain axis has grown from nothing to an established, growing body of knowledge. Gluten, the way it affects the gut, and the ongoing consequences has become critical in understanding many health issues. This is very good news. It could be the key to your own recovery.

Science and Specifics

More and more research and information is coming out linking brain and digestive track health. There are two main related aspects of the intestinal tract involved, gut permeability and the microbiome. Volumes have been written about this. I will try to keep it simple.

Gut permeability is how easy it is for molecules to go from inside your intestines into your blood stream. When food is digested it should be broken down into its basic parts, relatively small molecules. Then these are selectively allowed into your blood stream. If your gut is too permeable, larger molecules go through. This is known as leaky gut syndrome.

After those larger molecules escape the intestine, they're identified as foreign by the immune system. Antibodies are made against them and they are attacked. This process creates inflammation, which can, in turn, increase brain inflammation. Some leaky gut symptoms are also concussion symptoms: brain fog, fatigue, headaches. This makes it hard to know if the cause of the symptoms is the concussion or leaky gut. Other symptoms may include chronic diarrhea, constipation, bloating, joint pain, and skin problems. Specific digestive enzymes can be taken with meals to help break down the larger molecules before they have a chance to pass through the gut barrier. This may reduce the inflammatory load on the body and symptoms creating a window of opportunity for other healing. However, it does not address the underlying problem of permeability. Since gut and brain barrier permeability are related, it is essential to really get to the root cause and heal the gut.

Another issue that may occur is Small Intestinal Bacterial Overgrowth, (SIBO). This is when bacteria that are only supposed to live in the large intestine start getting into the small intestine. People with head injury are somewhat more susceptible to this because the movement of the bowels and the control of the valves in the digestive system are controlled by the Vagus nerve, a cranial nerve that originates in the brain stem. A key symptom of SIBO is bloating after meals. SIBO is a medical condition that will require testing to confirm. Treatment usually includes the use of antibiotics and a restrictive diet. Vagus nerve stimulation can also be helpful.

The greatest danger of leaky gut is the development of autoimmunity. This happens when the immune system produces antibodies for a foreign substance that resembles part of your own body and the immune system attacks both. Parts of the brain are vulnerable to this kind of autoimmunity; the most common example is the cerebellum, which can be mistaken as gluten. The cerebellum is responsible for balance, so balance problems can be caused by gluten-based autoimmunity. The medical term for this is gluten ataxia.

Many people have some degree of leaky gut that may or may not be symptomatic before a head injury. Even if you did not have leaky gut, it's been shown in mice that the gut barrier starts to break down in as little as 6.5 hours after a head trauma. [139]

The microbiome refers to bacteria, yeast, and viruses living in the intestines. Most of the research focuses on the bacteria, of which there are hundreds of types. Some are good for us. They help us break down food, process vitamins, or protect us from other bacteria which are bad for us. The balance and diversity of bacteria we have is important. When it's out of balance we call it dysbiosis. Symptoms of dysbiosis are the same as leaky gut and may include bloating or gas, particularly after eating a starchy meal. It's safe to say that those with frequent diarrhea or constipation, celiac disease, Crohn's disease, irritable bowel syndrome, or SIBO (Small Intestine Bacterial Overgrowth), also have dysbiosis. Dysbiosis contributes to brain inflammation.

Different bacteria feed on different plant fibers so we can support the diversity of our microbiome by eating a variety of plant fibers/vegetables. Soluble plant fiber is broken down by bacteria into short-chain fatty acids such as butyrate, which is used in many biological processes and as fuel for other gut bacteria. It also helps strengthen the gut barrier, making it less permeable. [140] Most importantly for the concussion patient, butyrate lessens microglial inflammatory action. [141] You can also supplement directly with short-chain fatty acids.

The microbiome can be harmed by alcohol, smoking, antibiotics, high-sugar foods, environmental toxins, stress, and lack of sleep or exercise. Of course, sometimes antibiotics are necessary, but if you need them, it's best to ask your doctor if you can take a targeted narrow- spectrum antibiotic versus a broad-spectrum antibiotic so fewer types of bacteria are killed. It's also helpful to supplement with probiotics, live bacteria, and yeast, to replenish the gut flora.

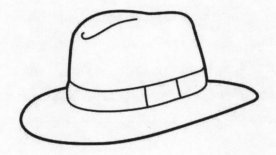

Part 8

Where to Go from Here

Summary

This book has been about creating a stable environment and the essential building blocks for your brain to heal. It's a process that takes time and effort. If you have done the work, your efforts should have been rewarded by a decrease in symptoms and increases in function. If some symptoms linger, you may have specific areas of your brain that you need to rehabilitate. You can rehabilitate your brain by forming new connections, which, as discussed in earlier chapters, is called neuroplasticity. There are many ways to go about doing this depending on your needs.

What to Do

In Chapter 20, Know Your Now, we talked about writing down and tracking symptoms. I also recommended neuropsychological testing to provide a more objective measured analysis of brain function. If you did get tested and return to your neuropsychologist later, hopefully, many symptoms have lessened or resolved, and the follow-up testing shows vast improvement. Take another look, however, and see where you still need to heal. Get help from professionals specializing in the resolution of those symptoms.

Why

When your brain is injured, it wants to heal. As you reduce and manage brain inflammation, control blood sugar, and heal your gut, nerves will form many new connections. Restoring blood flow to your brain and gradually challenging your brain to perform also aid in forming new nerve connections. You can regain a lot of lost function naturally through these processes. That being said, you may need more targeted therapies to stimulate specific areas of the brain to form new connections related to specific functions.

Personal Reflections

As discussed earlier in the book, to heal your brain, you must dampen the fire of neuroinflammation first. The flames cannot always be completely extinguished; sometimes they can only be managed, flaring up when that management fails. You may need to start developing new nerve connections while there's still some inflammation. Sometimes the act of developing new connections, itself, will also help lessen the smoldering.

Many different therapies are powerful means of recovery for the post-concussion patients, and they all address the causes of the symptoms they aim to resolve. One of these is vestibular therapy.

I had one patient who travelled a great distance for many months to get vestibular therapy without first addressing brain inflammation. This particular method involved sitting in a chair inside a kind of gyroscope that could move her body in any direction as she visually tracked a light. The practice provided her vestibular system with enormous amounts of stimulus and did create measurable improvement in balance. In that respect, it was working, and she did not want to give it up or take a break. The thing is, each time she did the therapy, the drive, the amount of stimulation, and the physical movement of her brain in her skull fatigued her brain and triggered more inflammation. It's impossible to say what could have been, but I believe that if she had done this same therapy after getting her brain inflammation to a manageable level, she would've gotten much better results.

Science and Specifics

Depending on your concussion symptoms, you may need help from one or more of the following provider types, listed below with the symptoms they treat:

Cognitive behavioral therapist - emotional volatility, depression, anxiety

Eye movement desensitization and reprocessing therapy (EMDR) - post-traumatic stress disorder (PTSD)

Occupational therapist - cognitive endurance, planning and pacing, balance and coordination issues, visual issues, sensory overload

Speech pathologist - speaking, swallowing, word finding. Memory, problem solving, planning, and attention as they relate to language.

Neuro-acupuncture - brain inflammation and oxygenation-related symptoms, difficulty transitioning out of the fight-flight mode. Helps stimulate neuroplasticity.

Neuro-physical therapy - balance and coordination as it relates to the integration of the body with the vestibular and visual systems.

Vestibular therapy - balance and coordination as it relates to the integration of the vestibular system with the body and visual systems.

Neuro-optometry - balance, coordination as it relates to the integration of the visual system with the body and vestibular systems. Visual disturbances, double vision, visual tracking issues.

Functional medicine - supporting any of the above through targeted neurotransmitter support.

Chapter 39

Moving Forward

Whether you've been dealing with concussion issues for one month or decades, you know there are good days and bad days. Some say the key is to accept your new self as you are. Others say the most important thing is to never give up. I say both are true.

People tend to have a fixed sense of who they are because they change slowly. We sense a continuity stretching back as far as we can remember leading to where we are today. That is what defines us. Head injury can change us so dramatically that it breaks that continuity. We are not "the person we used to be" and so we no longer know ourselves.

The natural desire is to go back to being the self we knew. We want to feel the same way we did then. Do the things we enjoyed. Think clearly. But we've been taken so off course that it may not be possible to go back. We have a new starting point. That much, I think we need to accept, but that doesn't mean staying there.

I once had a very kind teacher in Japan. I was interested in Buddhism and she was a nun. When I had trouble meditating, she assured me that I was perfect at every step of the path. I think this means we are right where we need to be right now. It allows us to take the next step, where we will also be perfect in that moment. Where or if we will arrive somewhere else is unknown. We need to stay on the path and appreciate each step. It's pointless to judge yourself or your situation when you and that situation are changing from moment to moment, day to day. You may never be the person you were before your head injury, but that's alright. We are always changing. No one is really the person they were yesterday.

As you move through your post-concussion life you will have many failures and many victories. Since there is no one solution to healing for anyone, both your failures and victories will be unique. They are yours. Appreciate what you learn from both.

With most health issues there is a beginning, middle, and end. The end is either full healing or ongoing management. With post-concussion syndrome, you may or may not get to that sense of end.

Please do not look at any one strategy as a cure. If you do, you will be disappointed and go from one strategy or practitioner to another with no satisfaction. What does not feel helpful for you now may be helpful at a later stage of healing and vice versa. If you look at each strategy as a piece of your own unique healing puzzle and keep each one that helps, you will make progress. All of these strategies tend to work better in combination. You need to find your own recipe for maximum recovery.

No matter what degree of recovery you reach, your life will have been greatly changed. You may always feel tension between wanting to be like you were and how you are now. As you become able to resume some activities, it's important to continue the healthy lifestyle changes that enabled you to do them. Many of the strategies discussed in this book are neuro-protective so, if you have another injury, it will be less severe than it might have been.

Remember you are on a path. Keep going. Be ever hopeful.

Wear a Hat

References

[1] Maas, Andrew IR, David K. Menon, Geoffrey T. Manley, Mathew Abrams, Cecilia Åkerlund, Nada Andelic, Marcel Aries et al. "Traumatic brain injury: progress and challenges in prevention, clinical care, and research." The Lancet Neurology (2022).

[2] Link, Jared S., Trevor Barker, Sophia Serpa, Maya Pinjala, Thomas Oswald, and Lisa K. Lashley. "Mild traumatic brain injury and mindfulness-based stress reduction: a review." Archives of assessment psychology 6, no. 1 (2016): 7-32.

[3] Kharrazian, Datis. Why isn't my brain working?. Elephant Press, 2013, p. 206-7.

[4] McClincy, MC and Lovell MR, Pardini J, Collins MW, Spore MK. Recovery from sports concussion in high school and collegiate athletes. Brain Injury. 2006;20(1):33–39.

[5] Maas, Andrew IR, David K. Menon, Geoffrey T. Manley, Mathew Abrams, Cecilia Åkerlund, Nada Andelic, Marcel Aries et al. "Traumatic brain injury: progress and challenges in prevention, clinical care, and research." The Lancet Neurology (2022).

[6] Varatharaj, Aravinthan, and Ian Galea. "The blood-brain barrier in systemic inflammation." Brain, behavior, and immunity 60 (2017): 1-12.

[7] Patterson, Zachary, Holahan Matthew. Understanding the neuroinflammatory response following concussion to develop treatment strategies. Frontiers in Cellular Neuroscience, Vol.6 2012, p58. DOI=10.3389/fncel.2012.00058

[8] Heyer MD, Geoffrey, Syed A.Idris MDDoes Analgesic Overuse Contribute to Chronic Post-traumatic Headaches in Adolescent Concussion Patients? Pediatric Neurology Volume 50, Issue 5, May 2014, Pages 464-468. https://doi.org/10.1016/j.pediatrneurol.2014.01.040

[9] K.D. Brown, Iwata, A., Putt, M.E., & Smith, D.H. (2006). Chronic ibuprophen administration worsens cognitive outcome following traumatic brain injury in rats. Experimental Neurology, 201(2), 301-307.doi:10.1016/j.expneurol.2006.04.008

[10] Petrelli MN NP PhD,Tina, Forough Farrokhyar, MPhil PhD, Patricia McGrath, PhD, Chris Sulowski, MD FRCPC, Gita Sobhi, BA BSc PHM, Carol DeMatteo, MSc Dip.P&OT, Lucia Giglia, BSc MSc MD FRCPC(C), Sheila K. Singh, MD PhD FRCSC, The use of ibuprofen and acetaminophen for acute headache in the postconcussive youth: A pilot study, Paediatrics & Child Health, Volume 22, Issue 1, 1 March 2017, Pages 2–6, https://doi.org/10.1093/pch/pxw011

[11] Bombardier, C.H., C.T. Rimmele & H. Zintel. 2002. The magnitude and correlates of alcohol and drug use before traumatic brain injury. Arch. Phys. Med. Rehabil. 83: 1765–1773.

[12] West, Steven L. 'Substance Use Among Persons with Traumatic Brain Injury: A Review'. 1 Jan. 2011: 1 – 8.

[13] Fann, J.R., Burington, B., Leonetti, A., Jaffe, K., Katon, W.J., and Thompson, R.S. (2004). Psychiatric illness following traumatic brain injury in an adult health maintenance organization population. Arch. Gen. Psychiatry 61, 53–61.

[14] Bjork, James M. and Steven J. Grant. Does Traumatic Brain Injury Increase Risk for Substance Abuse?. Journal of Neurotrauma 2009 26:7, 1077-1082.

[15] Fernández-Checa JC, Kaplowitz N, García-Ruiz C, Colell A, Miranda M, Marí M, Ardite E, Morales A. GSH transport in mitochondria: defense against TNF-induced oxidative stress and alcohol-induced defect. Am J Physiol. 1997 Jul;273(1 Pt 1):G7-17. doi: 10.1152/ajpgi.1997.273.1.G7. PMID: 9252504.

[16] Dai, Shuang-Shuang, Yuan-Guo Zhou, Wei Li, Jian-Hong An, Ping Li, Nan Yang, Xing-Yun Chen et al. "Local glutamate level dictates adenosine A2A receptor regulation of neuroinflammation and traumatic brain injury." Journal of Neuroscience 30, no. 16 (2010): 5802-5810.

[17] Petraglia AL, Winkler EA, Bailes JE. Stuck at the bench: Potential natural neuroprotective compounds for concussion. Surg Neurol Int. 2011;2:146. doi: 10.4103/2152-7806.85987. Epub 2011 Oct 12. PMID: 22059141; PMCID: PMC3205506.

[18] Alasmari, Fawaz. "Caffeine induces neurobehavioral effects through modulating neurotransmitters." Saudi Pharmaceutical Journal 28, no. 4 (2020): 445-451.

[19] White BC, Lincoln CA, Pearce NW, Reeb R, Vaida C. Anxiety and muscle tension as consequences of caffeine withdrawal. Science. 1980 Sep 26;209(4464):1547-8. DOI: 10.1126/science.7433978

[20] Ledesma ALL, Barreto MASC, Bahmad JR F. Caffeine effect in vestibular system. Int Tinnitus J. 2014;19(1):77-81

[21] Prajapati, Santosh Kumar, Durgesh Singh Dangi, and Sairam Krishnamurthy. "Repeated caffeine administration aggravates post-traumatic stress disorder-like symptoms in rats." Physiology & behavior 211 (2019): 112666.

[22] Lovallo WR, Whitsett TL, al'Absi M, Sung BH, Vincent AS, Wilson MF. Caffeine stimulation of cortisol secretion across the waking hours in relation to caffeine intake levels. Psychosom Med. 2005 Sep-Oct;67(5):734-9. doi: 10.1097/01.psy.0000181270.20036.06. PMID: 16204431; PMCID: PMC2257922.

[23] Durazzo, Timothy C., Linda Abadjian, Adam Kincaid, Tobias Bilovsky-Muniz, Lauren Boreta, and Grant E. Gauger The Influence of Chronic Cigarette Smoking on Neurocognitive Recovery after Mild Traumatic Brain Injury. Journal of Neurotrauma 2013 30:11, 1013-1022

[24] Grundey, Jessica, Nivethida Thirugnanasambandam, Kim Kaminsky, Anne Drees, Angela C. Skwirba, Nicolas Lang, Walter Paulus and Michael A. Nitsche Neuroplasticity in Cigarette Smokers Is Altered under Withdrawal and Partially Restituted by Nicotine Exposition Journal of Neuroscience 21 March 2012, 32 (12) 4156-4162; DOI: https://doi.org/10.1523/JNEUROSCI.3660-11.2012

[25] Durazzo, Timothy C., Linda Abadjian, Adam Kincaid, Tobias Bilovsky-Muniz, Lauren Boreta, and Grant E. Gauger The Influence of Chronic Cigarette Smoking on Neurocognitive Recovery after Mild Traumatic Brain Injury. Journal of Neurotrauma 2013 30:11, 1013-1022

[26] Roach, Sean P, ATC, CSCS, Megan N Houston, PhD, ATC, Karen Y Peck, MEd, ATC, CCRP, Steven J Svoboda, MC USA, (Ret.), MD, Tim F Kelly, MS, ATC, Steven R Malvasi, MS, ATC, Gerald T McGinty, BSC USAF, (Ret.), PT, DPT, Darren E Campbell, MC USAF, (Ret.), MD, Kenneth L Cameron, PhD, MPH, ATC, The Influence of Self-Reported Tobacco Use on Baseline Concussion Assessments, Military Medicine, Volume 185, Issue 3-4, March-April 2020, Pages e431–e437, https://doi.org/10.1093/milmed/usz352

[27] Durazzo, Timothy C., Dieter J. Meyerhoff, and Donna E. Murray 2015. "Comparison of Regional Brain Perfusion Levels in

Chronically Smoking and Non-Smoking Adults" International Journal of Environmental Research and Public Health 12, no. 7: 8198-8213. https://doi.org/10.3390/ijerph120708198

[28] Durazzo, Timothy C., Dieter J. Meyerhoff, and Sara Jo Nixon. 2010. "Chronic Cigarette Smoking: Implications for Neurocognition and Brain Neurobiology" International Journal of Environmental Research and Public Health 7, no. 10: 3760-3791. https://doi.org/10.3390/ijerph7103760

[29] Gallant C, Luczon R, Ryan D, Good D. Investigating cannabis use and associated symptoms among university students with and without a history of concussion. Neuropsychol Rehabil. 2020 Nov 18:1-25. doi: 10.1080/09602011.2020.1847148. Epub ahead of print. PMID: 33208035.

[30] Pope, Harrison G. and Deborah A. Yurgelun-Todd. "The residual cognitive effects of heavy marijuana use in college students." JAMA 275 7 (1996): 521-7.

[31] Ashton, C. H. Adverse effects of cannabis and cannabinoids. British Journal of Anaesthesia 83 (4): 637–49 (1999)

[32] Wu T-C, Tashkin DP, Djahed B, Rose JE. Pulmonary hazards of smoking marijuana as compared with tobacco. N Engl J Med 1988; 318: 347–51

[33] Gedin F, Blomé S, Pontén M, et al. Placebo Response and Media Attention in Randomized Clinical Trials Assessing Cannabis-Based Therapies for Pain: A Systematic Review and Meta-analysis. JAMA Netw Open. 2022;5(11):e2243848. doi:10.1001/jamanetworkopen.2022.43848

[34] Fishbein-Kaminietsky, M., Gafni, M. and Sarne, Y. (2014), Ultralow doses of cannabinoid drugs protect the mouse brain from inflammation-induced cognitive damage. Journal of Neuroscience Research, 92: 1669-1677. https://doi.org/10.1002/jnr.23452

[35] Rao, Vani, and Constantine Lyketsos. "Neuropsychiatric sequelae of traumatic brain injury." Psychosomatics 41, no. 2 (2000): 95-103.

[36] Lombard, Lisa A., and Ross D. Zafonte. "Agitation after traumatic brain injury: considerations and treatment options." American journal of physical medicine & rehabilitation 84, no. 10 (2005): 797-812.

[37] Hart T, Brockway JA, Maiuro RD, Vaccaro M, Fann JR, Mellick D, Harrison-Felix C, Barber J, Temkin N. Anger Self-Management Training for Chronic Moderate to Severe Traumatic Brain Injury: Results of a Randomized Controlled Trial. J Head Trauma Rehabil. 2017 Sep/Oct;32(5):319-331. doi: 10.1097/HTR.0000000000000316. PMID: 28520666; PMCID: PMC5593756.

[38] Lombard, Lisa A., and Ross D. Zafonte. "Agitation after traumatic brain injury: considerations and treatment options." American journal of physical medicine & rehabilitation 84, no. 10 (2005): 797-812.

[39] Volkow, N. D., G. J. Wang, J. Logan, D. Alexoff, J. S. Fowler, P. K. Thanos, C. Wong, V. Casado, S. Ferre, and D. Tomasi. "Caffeine increases striatal dopamine D2/D3 receptor availability in the human brain." Translational psychiatry 5, no. 4 (2015): e549-e549.

[40] Alasmari, Fawaz. "Caffeine induces neurobehavioral effects through modulating neurotransmitters." Saudi Pharmaceutical Journal 28, no. 4 (2020): 445-451.

[41] Acabchuk, R.L., Brisson, J.M., Park, C.L., Babbott-Bryan, N., Parmelee, O.A. and Johnson, B.T. (2021), Therapeutic Effects of Meditation, Yoga, and Mindfulness-Based Interventions for Chronic Symptoms of Mild Traumatic Brain Injury: A Systematic Review and Meta-Analysis. Appl Psychol Health Well-Being, 13: 34-62. https://doi.org/10.1111/aphw.12244

[42] Bramley H, Henson A, Lewis MM, Kong L, Stetter C, Silvis M. Sleep Disturbance Following Concussion Is a Risk Factor for a Prolonged Recovery. Clinical Pediatrics. 2017;56(14):1280-1285. doi:10.1177/0009922816681603

[43] Parsons, L. C., & ver Beek, D. (1982). Sleep-awake patterns following cerebral concussion. Nursing Research, 31(5), 260–264. https://doi.org/10.1097/00006199-198231050-00002

[44] Mihalik, Jason P. PhD*,†,‡; Lengas, Eric MA*; Register-Mihalik, Johna K. PhD§; Oyama, Sakiko PhD¶; Begalle, Rebecca L. MS†; Guskiewicz, Kevin M. PhD*,†,‡ The Effects of Sleep Quality and Sleep Quantity on Concussion Baseline Assessment, Clinical Journal of Sport Medicine: September 2013 - Volume 23 - Issue 5 - p 343-348 doi: 10.1097/JSM.0b013e318295a834

[45] Bramley H, Henson A, Lewis MM, Kong L, Stetter C, Silvis M. Sleep Disturbance Following Concussion Is a Risk Factor for a

Prolonged Recovery. Clinical Pediatrics. 2017;56(14):1280-1285.
doi:10.1177/0009922816681603

[46] Raikes, MS, LAT, ATC, Adam C., Sydney Y. Schaefer, PhD,
Sleep Quantity and Quality during Acute Concussion: A Pilot Study,
Sleep, Volume 39, Issue 12, 1 December 2016, Pages 2141–2147,
https://doi.org/10.5665/sleep.6314

[47] Thomasy, H., and M. Opp. "0278 HYPOCRETIN AS A
MEDIATOR OF POST-TRAUMATIC BRAIN INJURY SLEEP
DISTURBANCE." Sleep 40 (2017): A102.

[48] Wisor, Jonathan P., PhD, Michelle A. Schmidt, MS, William C.
Clegern, BS, Evidence for Neuroinflammatory and Microglial Changes in
the Cerebral Response to Sleep Loss, Sleep, Volume 34, Issue 3, March
2011, Pages 261–272, https://doi.org/10.1093/sleep/34.3.261

[49] Harrison, Jordan L., Rachel K. Rowe, Timothy W. Ellis, Nicole
S. Yee, Bruce F. O'Hara, P. David Adelson, Jonathan Lifshitz, Resolvins
AT-D1 and E1 differentially impact functional outcome, post-traumatic
sleep, and microglial activation following diffuse brain injury in the
mouse, Brain, Behavior, and Immunity, Volume 47, 2015, Pages 131-
140, ISSN 0889-1591, https://doi.org/10.1016/j.bbi.2015.01.001.

[50] Arita, Makoto, Francesca Bianchini, Julio Aliberti, Alan Sher,
Nan Chiang, Song Hong, Rong Yang, Nicos A. Petasis, Charles N.
Serhan; Stereochemical assignment, antiinflammatory properties, and
receptor for the omega-3 lipid mediator resolvin E1 . J Exp Med 7 March
2005; 201 (5): 713–722. doi: https://doi.org/10.1084/jem.20042031

[51] Rigon, Arianna , Nathaniel B. Klooster, Samantha Crooks and
Melissa C. Duff Severe Traumatic Brain Injury: Group Performance and
Individual Differences on the Rotary Pursuit Task Front. Hum. Neurosci.,
19 July 2019 https://doi.org/10.3389/fnhum.2019.00251

[52] Vakil, Eli (2005) The Effect of Moderate to Severe Traumatic
Brain Injury (TBI) on Different Aspects of Memory: A Selective Review,
Journal of Clinical and Experimental Neuropsychology, 27:8, 977-1021,
DOI: 10.1080/13803390490919245

[53] Pessoa, Luiz, Sabine Kastner, Leslie G. Ungerleider
Neuroimaging Studies of Attention: From Modulation of Sensory
Processing to Top-Down Control Journal of Neuroscience 15 May 2003,
23 (10) 3990-3998; DOI: 10.1523/JNEUROSCI.23-10-03990.2003

[54] Sudimac, Sonja, Vera Sale, and Simone Kühn. "How nature nurtures: Amygdala activity decreases as the result of a one-hour walk in nature." (2022).

[55] Rink, Cameron, and Savita Khanna. "Significance of brain tissue oxygenation and the arachidonic acid cascade in stroke." Antioxidants & redox signaling 14, no. 10 (2011): 1889-1903.

[56] Gray, Bruce G., Masanori Ichise, Dae-Gyun Chung, Joel C. Kirsh, and William Franks. "Technetium-99m-HMPAO SPECT in the evaluation of patients with a remote history of traumatic brain injury: a comparison with x-ray computed tomography." Journal of Nuclear Medicine 33, no. 1 (1992): 52-58.

[57] Krishnamoorthy V, Chaikittisilpa N, Kiatchai T, Vavilala M. Hypertension After Severe Traumatic Brain Injury: Friend or Foe? J Neurosurg Anesthesiol. 2017 Oct;29(4):382-387. doi: 10.1097/ANA.0000000000000370. PMID: 27648804; PMCID: PMC5357208.

[58] Boussi-Gross, Rahav, Haim Golan, Gregori Fishlev, Yair Bechor, Olga Volkov, Jacob Bergan, Mony Friedman et al. "Hyperbaric oxygen therapy can improve post concussion syndrome years after mild traumatic brain injury-randomized prospective trial." PloS one 8, no. 11 (2013): e79995.

[59] Yoon KJ, Kim DY. Immediate Effects of a Single Exercise on Behavior and Memory in the Early Period of Traumatic Brain Injury in Rats. Ann Rehabil Med. 2018;42(5):643–651. doi:10.5535/arm.2018.42.5.643

[60] Spielman, Lindsay Joy, Jonathan PeterLittle, Andis Klegerisa. Physical activity and exercise attenuate neuroinflammation in neurological diseases. Brain Research Bulletin, Volume 125, July 2016, Pages 19-29. https://doi.org/10.1016/j.brainresbull.2016.03.012

[61] Jelleyman, C., Yates, T., O'Donovan, G., Gray, L.J., King, J.A., Khunti, K. and Davies, M.J. (2015), The effects of HIIT on metabolic health. Obes Rev, 16: 942-961. doi:10.1111/obr.12317

[62] Prins, Mayumi L and Joyce H. Matsumoto. The collective therapeutic potential of cerebral ketone metabolism in traumatic brain injury. Journal of Lipid Research 55 (2014): 2450-2457. Https://doi.org/10.1194/jlr.R046706.

[63] Shi, J., Dong, B., Mao, Y., Guan, W., Cao, J., Zhu, R., & Wang, S. (2016). Review: Traumatic brain injury and hyperglycemia, a potentially modifiable risk factor. Oncotarget, 7(43), 71052–71061. https://doi.org/10.18632/oncotarget.11958

[64] Sekar S, Viswas RS, Miranzadeh Mahabadi H, Alizadeh E, Fonge H, Taghibiglou C. Concussion/Mild Traumatic Brain Injury (TBI) Induces Brain Insulin Resistance: A Positron Emission Tomography (PET) Scanning Study. Int J Mol Sci. 2021 Aug 20;22(16):9005. doi: 10.3390/ijms22169005. PMID: 34445708; PMCID: PMC8396497.

[65] Kharrazian, Why isn't my brain working?, 71-77.

[66] Gilsanz P, Albers K, Beeri MS, Karter AJ, Quesenberry CP Jr, Whitmer RA. Traumatic brain injury associated with dementia risk among people with type 1 diabetes. *Neurology*. 2018;91(17):e1611–e1618.

[67] Ley EJ, Srour MK, Clond MA, Barnajian M, Tillou A, Mirocha J, Salim A. Diabetic patients with traumatic brain injury: insulin deficiency is associated with increased mortality. J Trauma. 2011 May;70(5):1141-4. doi: 10.1097/TA.0b013e3182146d66. PMID: 21610428.

[68] Ley EJ, Srour MK, Clond MA, Barnajian M, Tillou A, Mirocha J, Salim A. Diabetic patients with traumatic brain injury: insulin deficiency is associated with increased mortality. J Trauma. 2011 May;70(5):1141-4. doi: 10.1097/TA.0b013e3182146d66. PMID: 21610428.

[69] Po-Chiao Chang, et al. Advanced glycosylation end products induce inducible nitric oxide synthase (iNOS) expression via a p38 MAPK-dependent pathway. Kidney International Volume 65, Issue 5, May 2004, Pages 1664-1675. https://doi.org/10.1111/j.1523-1755.2004.00602.x

[70] Takeda, A., Yasuda, T., Miyata, T. et al. Advanced glycation end products co-localized with astrocytes and microglial cells in Alzheimer's disease brain Acta Neuropathol (1998) 95: 555. https://doi.org/10.1007/s004010050839

[71] Barbagallo M, Dominguez LJ. Magnesium and type 2 diabetes. *World J Diabetes*. 2015;6(10):1152–1157. doi:10.4239/wjd.v6.i10.1152

[72] Shukla, AP, Dickison, M, Coughlin, N, et al. The impact of food order on postprandial glycaemic excursions in prediabetes. Diabetes Obes Metab. 2019; 21: 377– 381. https://doi.org/10.1111/dom.13503

[73] Z. Z. X. Leow,K. J. Guelfi,E. A. Davis,T. W. Jones,P. A. Fournier. The glycaemic benefits of a very-low-carbohydrate ketogenic diet in adults with Type 1 diabetes mellitus may be opposed by increased hypoglycaemia risk and dyslipidaemia. Diabetic Medicine Volume35, Issue9 September 2018 Pages 1258-1263. https://doi.org/10.1111/dme.13663

[74] Prins, Mayumi L and Joyce H. Matsumoto. The collective therapeutic potential of cerebral ketone metabolism in traumatic brain injury. Journal of Lipid Research 55 (2014): 2450-2457. Https://doi.org/10.1194/jlr.R046706.

[75] Nicole J.Jensen, Helena Z. Wodschow, Malin Nilsson, and Jørgen Rungby. 2020. Effects of Ketone Bodies on Brain Metabolism and Function in Neurodegenerative Diseases International Journal of Molecular Sciences 21, no. 22: 8767. https://doi.org/10.3390/ijms21228767

[76] Mark F McCarty and Aaron Lerner. The second phase of brain trauma can be controlled by nutraceuticals that suppress DAMP-mediated microglial activation Expert Review of Neurotherapeutics, 21:5, 559-570, (2021) DOI: 10.1080/14737175.2021.1907182

[77] Liśkiewicz, D., Liskiewicz, A., Nowacka-Chmielewska, M., Student, S., Anna, S., Konstancja, J., . . . Małecki, A. (2020). Brain macroautophagy on the ketogenic diet. Proceedings of the Nutrition Society, 79(OCE2), E235. doi:10.1017/S0029665120001834

[78] Ma, D., Wang, A.C., Parikh, I. et al. Ketogenic diet enhances neurovascular function with altered gut microbiome in young healthy mice. Sci Rep 8, 6670 (2018). https://doi.org/10.1038/s41598-018-25190-5

[79] ST Henderson. Ketone bodies as a therapeutic for Alzheimer's disease. Neurotherapeutics. 2008 Jul;5(3):470-80. doi: 10.1016/j.nurt.2008.05.004. PMID: 18625458; PMCID: PMC5084248.

[80] Francis N. Intermittent Fasting and Brain Health: Efficacy and Potential Mechanisms of Action. OBM Geriatrics 2020; 4(2): 121; doi:10.21926/obm.geriatr.2002121.

[81] A. Wu, Z.Yinga, F.Gomez-Pinilla. Exercise facilitates the action of dietary DHA on functional recovery after brain trauma, Neuroscience Volume 248, 17 September 2013, Pages 655-663.

[82] Aiguo Wu, Zhe Ying, and Fernando Gomez-Pinilla. Dietary Omega-3 Fatty Acids Normalize BDNF Levels, Reduce Oxidative Damage, and Counteract Learning Disability after Traumatic Brain Injury in Rats, Journal of Neurotrauma 2004 21:10, 1457-1467

[83] Mills, James D., Kevin Hadley, Julian E. Bailes, Dietary Supplementation With the Omega-3 Fatty Acid Docosahexaenoic Acid in Traumatic Brain Injury, Neurosurgery, Volume 68, Issue 2, February 2011, Pages 474–481, https://doi.org/10.1227/NEU.0b013e3181ff692b

[84] Hasadsri, Linda, Bonnie H. Wang, James V. Lee, John W. Erdman, Daniel A. Llano, Aron K. Barbey, Tracey Wszalek, Matthew F. Sharrock, and Huan (John) Wang. Omega-3 Fatty Acids as a Putative Treatment for Traumatic Brain InjuryJournal of Neurotrauma.Jun 2013.897-906.http://doi.org/10.1089/neu.2012.2672

[85] Harvey LD, Yin Y, Attarwala IY, et al. Administration of DHA Reduces Endoplasmic Reticulum Stress-Associated Inflammation and Alters Microglial or Macrophage Activation in Traumatic Brain Injury. ASN Neuro. December 2015. doi:10.1177/1759091415618969

[86] Charrière, Karine, Imen Ghzaiel, Gérard Lizard, and Anne Vejux. 2021. "Involvement of Microglia in Neurodegenerative Diseases: Beneficial Effects of Docosahexahenoic Acid (DHA) Supplied by Food or Combined with Nanoparticles" International Journal of Molecular Sciences 22, no. 19: 10639. https://doi.org/10.3390/ijms221910639

[87] Aiguo Wu, Zhe Ying, and Fernando Gomez-Pinilla.The Salutary Effects of DHA Dietary Supplementation on Cognition, Neuroplasticity, and Membrane Homeostasis after Brain TraumaJournal of Neurotrauma.Oct 2011. 2113-2122. http://doi.org/10.1089/neu.2011.1872

[88] Harrison, Jordan L., Rachel K. Rowe, Timothy W. Ellis, Nicole S. Yee, Bruce F. O'Hara, P. David Adelson, Jonathan Lifshitz, Resolvins AT-D1 and E1 differentially impact functional outcome, post-traumatic sleep, and microglial activation following diffuse brain injury in the mouse, Brain, Behavior, and Immunity, Volume 47, 2015, Pages 131-140, ISSN 0889-1591, https://doi.org/10.1016/j.bbi.2015.01.001.

[89] Arita, Makoto, Francesca Bianchini, Julio Aliberti, Alan Sher, Nan Chiang, Song Hong, Rong Yang, Nicos A. Petasis, Charles N. Serhan; Stereochemical assignment, antiinflammatory properties, and receptor for the omega-3 lipid mediator resolvin E1 . J Exp Med 7 March 2005; 201 (5): 713–722. doi: https://doi.org/10.1084/jem.20042031

[90] Byelashov OA, Sinclair AJ, Kaur G. Dietary sources, current intakes, and nutritional role of omega-3 docosapentaenoic acid. Lipid Technol. 2015;27(4):79–82. doi:10.1002/lite.201500013

[91] Mason RP, Sherratt SCR. Omega-3 fatty acid fish oil dietary supplements contain saturated fats and oxidized lipids that may interfere with their intended biological benefits. Biochem Biophys Res Commun. 2017 Jan 29;483(1):425-429. doi: 10.1016/j.bbrc.2016.12.127. Epub 2016 Dec 21. PMID: 28011269.

[92] U.S. Department of Agriculture, Agricultural Research Service. FoodData Central, 2019. fdc.nal.usda.gov. FDC ID: 171400 NDB Number:4001.

[93] U.S. Department of Agriculture, Agricultural Research Service. FoodData Central, 2019. fdc.nal.usda.gov. FDC ID: 343868 Food Code:82101500.

[94] Ginter E, Simko V. New data on harmful effects of trans-fatty acids. Bratisl Lek Listy. 2016;117(5):251–253. doi:10.4149/bll_2016_048

[95] Song J, Park J, Jung J, et al. Analysis of Trans Fat in Edible Oils with Cooking Process. Toxicol Res. 2015;31(3):307–312. doi:10.5487/TR.2015.31.3.307

[96]"Dietary Reference Intakes" Institute of Medicine of the National Acadamies 2005 https://www.nal.usda.gov/sites/default/files/fnic_uploads/energy_full_rep ort.pdf

[97] Gómez Candela C, Bermejo López LM, Loria Kohen V. Importance of a balanced omega 6/omega 3 ratio for the maintenance of health: nutritional recommendations. Nutr Hosp. 2011;26(2):323–329. doi:10.1590/S0212-16112011000200013

[98] Calder PC. Polyunsaturated fatty acids and inflammatory processes: New twists in an old tale. Biochimie. 2009;91(6):791–795. doi:10.1016/j.biochi.2009.01.008

[99] Andruchow, N. D., Konishi, K., Shatenstein, B., & Bohbot, V. D. (2017). A lower ratio of omega-6 to omega-3 fatty acids predicts better hippocampus-dependent spatial memory and cognitive status in older adults. Neuropsychology, 31(7), 724–734. https://doi.org/10.1037/neu0000373

[100] Loef M, Walach H. The omega-6/omega-3 ratio and dementia or cognitive decline: a systematic review on human studies and biological evidence. J Nutr Gerontol Geriatr. 2013;32(1):1–23. doi:10.1080/21551197.2012.752335

[101] Dumas, Julie A., Janice Y. Bunn, Joshua Nickerson, Karen I. Crain, David B. Ebenstein, Emily K. Tarleton, Jenna Makarewicz, Matthew E. Poynter, and Craig Lawrence Kien. "Dietary saturated fat and monounsaturated fat have reversible effects on brain function and the secretion of pro-inflammatory cytokines in young women." Metabolism 65, no. 10 (2016): 1582-1588.

[102] Wu, A., R. Molteni, Z. Ying, and F. Gomez-Pinilla. "A saturated-fat diet aggravates the outcome of traumatic brain injury on hippocampal plasticity and cognitive function by reducing brain-derived neurotrophic factor." Neuroscience 119, no. 2 (2003): 365-375.

[103] I Lingam and Robertson N, J: Magnesium as a Neuroprotective Agent: A Review of Its Use in the Fetus, Term Infant with Neonatal Encephalopathy, and the Adult Stroke Patient. Dev Neurosci 2018;40:1-12. doi: 10.1159/000484891

[104].McDonald, John W, Faye S.Silverstein,Michael V.Johnston Magnesium reduces N-methyl-D-aspartate (NMDA)-mediated brain injury in perinatal rats. DataNeuroscience letters, ISSN: 0304-3940, Vol: 109, Issue: 1-2, Page: 234-8 https://doi.org/10.1016/0304-3940(90)90569-U

[105] Vink,Robert -,Christine A.O'Connor, Alan J.Nimmo, Deanne L.Heath Magnesium attenuates persistent functional deficits following diffuse traumatic brain injury in rats. Neuroscience Letters Volume 336, Issue 1, 9 January 2003, Pages 41-44. https://doi.org/10.1016/S0304-3940(02)01244-2.

[106] Zhu D, Su Y, Fu B, Xu H. Magnesium Reduces Blood-Brain Barrier Permeability and Regulates Amyloid-β Transcytosis. Mol Neurobiol. 2018 Sep;55(9):7118-7131. doi: 10.1007/s12035-018-0896-0. Epub 2018 Jan 30. PMID: 29383689.

[107] Hardwick, Laurie L., et al. Magnesium Absorption: Mechanisms and the Influence of Vitamin D, Calcium and Phosphate, The Journal of Nutrition, Volume 121, Issue 1, January 1991, Pages 13–23, https://doi.org/10.1093/jn/121.1.13

[108] Casazza K, Swanson E. Nutrition as Medicine to Improve Outcomes in Adolescents Sustaining a Sports-related

Concussion. *Explor Res Hypothesis Med*. 2017;2(4):122. doi: 10.14218/ERHM.2017.00029.

[109] Lawrence, David W. & Bhanu Sharma (2016) A review of the neuroprotective role of vitamin D in traumatic brain injury with implications for supplementation post-concussion, Brain Injury, 30:8, 960-968, DOI: 10.3109/02699052.2016.1147081

[110] Lawrence D. et al. Vitamin D Hormone Confers Neuroprotection in Parallel with Downregulation of L-Type Calcium Channel Expression in Hippocampal Neurons Journal of Neuroscience 1 January 2001, 21 (1) 98-108; DOI: 10.1523/JNEUROSCI.21-01-00098.2001

[111] Boontanrart, Mandy, Samuel D. Hall, Justin A. Spanier, Colleen E. Hayes, Julie K. Olson. Vitamin D3 alters microglia immune activation by an IL-10 dependent SOCS3 mechanism, Journal of Neuroimmunology 292 (2016) 126–136. https://doi.org/10.1016/j.jneuroim.2016.01.015

[112] Hardwick, Laurie L., Michael R. Jones, Nachman Brautbar, David B. N. Lee, Magnesium Absorption: Mechanisms and the Influence of Vitamin D, Calcium and Phosphate, The Journal of Nutrition, Volume 121, Issue 1, January 1991, Pages 13–23, https://doi.org/10.1093/jn/121.1.13

[113] Campos-Bedolla, P, Walter FR, Veszelka S, Deli MA. Role of the blood-brain barrier in the nutrition of the central nervous system. Arch Med Res. 2014;45(8):610-638. doi:10.1016/j.arcmed.2014.11.018

[114] Chen, Chong, Qingqing Ding, Boyu Shen, Tengjie Yu, He Wang, Yangfan Xu, Huimin Guo, Kangrui Hu, Lin Xie, Guangji Wang and Yan Liang Drug Metabolism and Disposition January 1, 2020, 48 (1) 52-62; DOI: https://doi.org/10.1124/dmd.119.089458

[115] Witschi A, Reddy S, Stofer B, Lauterburg BH. The systemic availability of oral glutathione. Eur J Clin Pharmacol. 1992;43(6):667-9. doi: 10.1007/BF02284971. PMID: 1362956.

[116] Sinha R, Sinha I, Calcagnotto A, Trushin N, Haley JS, Schell TD, Richie JP Jr. Oral supplementation with liposomal glutathione elevates body stores of glutathione and markers of immune function. Eur J Clin Nutr. 2018 Jan;72(1):105-111. doi: 10.1038/ejcn.2017.132. Epub 2017 Aug 30. PMID: 28853742; PMCID: PMC6389332.

[117] Vogel JU, Cinatl J, Dauletbaev N, Buxbaum S, Treusch G, Cinatl J Jr, Gerein V, Doerr HW. Effects of S-acetylglutathione in cell and animal model of herpes simplex virus type 1 infection. Med Microbiol Immunol. 2005 Jan;194(1-2):55-9. doi: 10.1007/s00430-003-0212-z. Epub 2003 Nov 18. PMID: 14624358.

[118] G. Courtney-Martin, P.B. Pencharz.The Molecular Nutrition of Amino Acids and Proteins, Sulfur Amino Acids Metabolism From Protein Synthesis to Glutathione. Academic Press, 2016, Pages 265-286.

[119] Petraglia AL, Winkler EA, Bailes JE. Stuck at the bench: Potential natural neuroprotective compounds for concussion. Surg Neurol Int. 2011;2:146. doi: 10.4103/2152-7806.85987. Epub 2011 Oct 12. PMID: 22059141; PMCID: PMC3205506.

[120] Rendeiro, Catarina, Justin S. Rhodes, and Jeremy PE Spencer. "The mechanisms of action of flavonoids in the brain: Direct versus indirect effects." Neurochemistry international 89 (2015): 126-139.

[121] Spagnuolo C, Moccia S, Russo GL. Anti-inflammatory effects of flavonoids in neurodegenerative disorders. Eur J Med Chem. 2018 Jun 10;153:105-115. doi: 10.1016/j.ejmech.2017.09.001. Epub 2017 Sep 7. PMID: 28923363.

[122] Kawabata, Kyuichi, Yasukiyo Yoshioka, and Junji Terao. 2019. "Role of Intestinal Microbiota in the Bioavailability and Physiological Functions of Dietary Polyphenols" Molecules 24, no. 2: 370. https://doi.org/10.3390/molecules24020370

[123] Frolinger, T., Sims, S., Smith, C. et al. The gut microbiota composition affects dietary polyphenols-mediated cognitive resilience in mice by modulating the bioavailability of phenolic acids. Sci Rep 9, 3546 (2019). https://doi.org/10.1038/s41598-019-39994-6

[124] Murphy L. Y Wan, Vanessa Anna Co & Hani El-Nezami (2021) Dietary polyphenol impact on gut health and microbiota, Critical Reviews in Food Science and Nutrition, 61:4, 690-711, DOI: 10.1080/10408398.2020.1744512

[125] Kam, Antony, K. M Li, Valentina Razmovski-Naumovski, Srinivas Nammi, Kelvin Chan, Yichiao Li, and G. Q Li. "The protective effects of natural products on blood-brain barrier breakdown." Current medicinal chemistry 19, no. 12 (2012): 1830-1845.

[126] Hsu, Cheng-Chin, Chien-Hsiang Cheng, Chin-Lin Hsu, Wan-Ju Lee, Shih-Chien Huang, and Yi-Chia Huang. "Role of vitamin B6 status on antioxidant defenses, glutathione, and related enzyme activities in mice with homocysteine-induced oxidative stress." Food & Nutrition Research 59, no. 1 (2015): 25702.

[127] Haar, Cole Vonder, Todd C. Peterson, Kris M. Martens, and Michael R. Hoane. "Vitamins and nutrients as primary treatments in experimental brain injury: Clinical implications for nutraceutical therapies." Brain research 1640 (2016): 114-129.

[128] Ambrogini, Patrizia, Pierangelo Torquato, Desirée Bartolini, Maria Cristina Albertini, Davide Lattanzi, Michael Di Palma, Rita Marinelli, Michele Betti, Andrea Minelli, Riccardo Cuppini, Francesco Galli. Excitotoxicity, neuroinflammation and oxidant stress as molecular bases of epileptogenesis and epilepsy-derived neurodegeneration: The role of vitamin E, Biochimica et Biophysica Acta (BBA) - Molecular Basis of Disease, Volume 1865, Issue 6, 2019, Pages 1098-1112, ISSN 0925-4439, https://doi.org/10.1016/j.bbadis.2019.01.026.

[129] La Torre, Maria Ester, Ines Villano, Marcellino Monda, Antonietta Messina, Giuseppe Cibelli, Anna Valenzano, Daniela Pisanelli, Maria Antonietta Panaro, Nicola Tartaglia, Antonio Ambrosi, Marco Carotenuto, Vincenzo Monda, Giovanni Messina, and Chiara Porro. 2021. "Role of Vitamin E and the Orexin System in Neuroprotection" Brain Sciences 11, no. 8: 1098. https://doi.org/10.3390/brainsci11081098

[130] Heppner, Frank L., Karl Roth, Robert Nitsch, and Nils P. Hailer. "Vitamin E induces ramification and downregulation of adhesion molecules in cultured microglial cells." Glia 22, no. 2 (1998): 180-188.

[131] Wenzel, Tyler J., Ellen J. Gates, Athena L. Ranger, and Andis Klegeris. "Short-chain fatty acids (SCFAs) alone or in combination regulate select immune functions of microglia-like cells." Molecular and Cellular Neuroscience 105 (2020): 103493.

[132] Li, Haonan, Yujiao Xiang, Zemeng Zhu, Wei Wang, Zhijun Jiang, Mingyue Zhao, Shuyue Cheng et al. "Rifaximin-Mediated Gut Microbiota Regulation Modulates the Polarization of Microglia During CUMS in Rat." (2021).

[133] Tuohy, Kieran M., Lorenza Conterno, Mattia Gasperotti, and Roberto Viola Up-regulating the Human Intestinal Microbiome Using

Whole Plant Foods, Polyphenols, and/or Fiber. Journal of Agricultural and Food Chemistry 2012 60 (36), 8776-8782 DOI: 10.1021/jf2053959

[134] Rathmacher, John A., John C. Fuller Jr, Shawn M. Baier, Naji N. Abumrad, Hector F. Angus, and Rick L. Sharp. "Adenosine-5'-triphosphate (ATP) supplementation improves low peak muscle torque and torque fatigue during repeated high intensity exercise sets." Journal of the International Society of Sports Nutrition 9, no. 1 (2012): 48.

[135] Singh, J., & Neary, J. (2020). Neuroprotection Following Concussion: The Potential Role for Cannabidiol. Canadian Journal of Neurological Sciences / Journal Canadien Des Sciences Neurologiques, 47(3), 289-300. doi:10.1017/cjn.2020.23

[136] Liem, Torsten. Cranial osteopathy. Philadelphia, PA: Churchill Livingstone, 2004, p 17-26.

[137] Marshall, Cameron M., Howard Vernon, John J. Leddy, and Bradley A. Baldwin. "The role of the cervical spine in post-concussion syndrome." The Physician and sportsmedicine 43, no. 3 (2015): 274-284.

[138] Liem, Torsten. Cranial osteopathy. Philadelphia, PA: Churchill Livingstone, 2004, p.2.

[139] Bansal,Vishal, Todd Costantini, Lauren Kroll, Carrie Peterson, William Loomis, Brian Eliceiri, Andrew Baird, Paul Wolf, and Raul Coimbra.Traumatic Brain Injury and Intestinal Dysfunction: Uncovering the Neuro-Enteric Axis.Journal of Neurotrauma.Aug 2009.1353-1359.http://doi.org/10.1089/neu.2008.0858

[140] Yan, Hui, and Kolapo M. Ajuwon. "Butyrate modifies intestinal barrier function in IPEC-J2 cells through a selective upregulation of tight junction proteins and activation of the Akt signaling pathway." PloS one 12, no. 6 (2017): e0179586.

[141] Matt, Stephanie M., Jacob M. Allen, Marcus A. Lawson, Lucy J. Mailing, Jeffrey A. Woods, and Rodney W. Johnson. "Butyrate and dietary soluble fiber improve neuroinflammation associated with aging in mice." Frontiers in immunology (2018): 1832.

Index

blood sugar, 221, 229–33
elimination, 301
ketogenic. *See* ketogenic
diet.
low-carb, 232, 234, 242,
248
digestive system, 282–83,
299–300, 305
disease, celiac, 302–3, 306
distractions, 158, 177
dizziness, 99, 195, 291–95,
300
doctors, 52, 289–90
homeopathic, 74–75, 209
medical, 83, 196, 209, 222
dopamine, 124, 146, 151, 226
drinking, 86, 91, 137, 234
drugs, 81, 85, 86, 110, 138
dura, 60, 290
dysbiosis, 299, 306
EMDR. *See* Eye Movement
Desensitization.
endocrine system, 222
energy, 59, 87, 158–61, 197,
264, 270, 273, 277–78
alcohol, 90
blood sugar, 211–34, 248
caffeine, 93–100
intermittent fasting, 248
ketogenic diet, 236–41
energy management, 46, 158
energy production, 92, 271
eNOS, 199, 277–78
EPA, 168, 250–57, 260
excitotoxicity. *See* neuro-
excitotoxicity.
executive function, 29, 42,
105–7, 123, 150

exercise, 139, 164, 195–206,
226–27, 249, 277–78, 307
cognitive, 57, 123, 158,
180, 207, 298
core, 206
high-intensity, 199–206
low-impact, 201–2
Eye Movement
Desensitization (EMDR),
126–27, 163, 312
fats, 193, 214, 218, 232–36,
241–43, 256–62
essential, 250–54
omega-3, 250–51, 255–
61
omega-6, 252, 257–61
mono-unsaturated, 261
Omega-6 and Omega-3
balance, 252–61
polyunsaturated, 257–60
saturated, 258–59, 261–62
fiber, 230, 238, 275–76, 306
fish oil supplements, 254,
271
flavonoids, 274–77
free radicals. *See* reactive
oxygen species (ROS).
functional dentists, 39, 292
functional medicine, 208–9,
222–23, 300, 313
Functional Reactive
Hypoglycemia, 224
glands
adrenal, 99, 199, 212–13,
216, 222, 231
pituitary, 222
glial cells. *See also* microglia
and astrocytes, 73, 272
glucose levels, 214, 218, 237

Made in the USA
Middletown, DE
08 December 2023

43887534R00208